Chronically Ill and At Risk Infants

Family-Centered Intervention from Hospital to Home

Kathy S. Katz, Ph.D.
Judith L. Pokorni, Ph.D.
Toby M. Long, M.A., P.T.

Georgetown University
Child Development Center

Published by:
VORT Corporation
Palo Alto, CA 94306

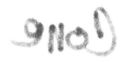

Published by:
  VORT Corporation
  PO Box 60132
  Palo Alto, CA 94306

ISBN 0-89718-121-2

CONTENTS

PREFACE

The authors of this guide began providing intensive intervention for chronically ill infants and their families as a part of the Chronically Ill Infant Intervention (CIII) Project begun in 1985. The CIII Project was developed through a Handicapped Children's Early Education Program grant from the U.S. Department of Education, Office of Special Education Programs, to the Georgetown University Child Development Center. The CIII Project provides services to chronically ill infants from shortly after birth until they are ready for transition into community based early intervention programs. The intervention is provided in three phases: Neonatal Intensive Care Unit (NICU), Home, and Pediatric Intensive Care Unit (PICU).

The experience of these years, including both successes and failures, forms the basis for the information presented in this guide. The guide begins with an overview of the CIII Project and its philosophy and continues with the critical information needed for an interdisciplinary team to design and implement an effective program for these special infants and their families. Because the program components are so interwoven, the authors recommend reading the complete guide before any one phase is implemented.

This guide is the result of the combined efforts of a number of Georgetown University Child Development Center staff. Other members of the CIII Project provided invaluable insight and expertise regarding the needs of chronically ill infants and their families. In particular, Maureen Reilly, M.S.N., C.P.N.P., nurse practitioner, and Cindy Baker, M.A., infant education specialist, showed unremitting patience and perseverance in their support of the CIII families. They also contributed in the development of several chapters of this guide. Brenda Hussey-Gardner, M.A., M.P.H., a member of our infant education staff, was responsible for preliminary drafts of several chapters. Her excellent knowledge of intervention in the NICU greatly enriched these sections. Other members of the Child Development Center especially Janet Thomas, O.T.R., Director of the Division of Occupational Therapy, contributed their time and expertise in working with our families. To these and all of our colleagues we extend our appreciation.

The outstanding drawings for the guide were executed by Dani LeMense, Laura Norden, and Melanie Snyder. Transcription of the guide was the effort of Vernice Thompson and Judy Kirk, for whose unflappable good humor we are all grateful.

We owe a great deal of thanks to the Georgetown University Hospital NICU staff, especially Janet Vail, R.N., Nursing Coordinator, and Dr. Sivasubramanian, Chief of the Neonatology Division. Their warm reception to the project was invaluable in garnering staff support.

Above all, we wish to express our gratitude to the CIII families for sharing their experiences with us and teaching us a great deal about the value and meaning of life with a chronically ill child.

Georgetown University
Child Development Center
Washington, D.C.

Kathy S. Katz
Project Director

Judith L. Pokorni
Project Coordinator

Toby M. Long
Director of Physical Therapy

1   THE CIII MODEL: AN OVERVIEW

Technological advances in the Neonatal Intensive Care Unit (NICU) have resulted in dramatically increased survival rates for low birthweight premature infants and other babies with major medical complications. While the prognosis to develop no major handicapping condition has increased for most NICU survivors, the estimate of major handicap for the smallest survivors remains about 30% (Hack and Fanaroff, 1986). These infants often remain medically fragile because of respiratory compromise, tracheostomies, gastrostomy tubes, severe seizure disorders, and other profound neurological damage.

The Georgetown University Child Development Center staff has become increasingly concerned about some of the children seen at the Developmental Evaluation Clinic (DEC). The clinic routinely assesses infants from the Georgetown University Hospital NICU during their first two years of life. The smallest survivors and others with chronic illnesses are often in need of developmental intervention. The focus on the medical needs of these infants, however, obscures the importance of the early years for cognitive, neuromotor, and psychosocial development. Because of chronic health conditions, these children are often unable to use community based developmental services: either they remain hospitalized, or are medically fragile, or their parents are preoccupied with necessary medical services. The clinic staff's concerns prompted the Child Development Center to propose the Chronically Ill Infant Intervention (CIII) Project. The CIII Project received funding in 1985 as a Handicapped Children's Early Education Program (HCEEP) from the U.S. Department of Education.

The CIII Project provides developmental intervention to chronically ill and medically fragile infants as well as support and training to parents in the understanding of the developmental needs of their infants. The Project consists of three interrelated components: **NICU, home,** and **Pediatric Intensive Care Unit (PICU)** [Figure 1].

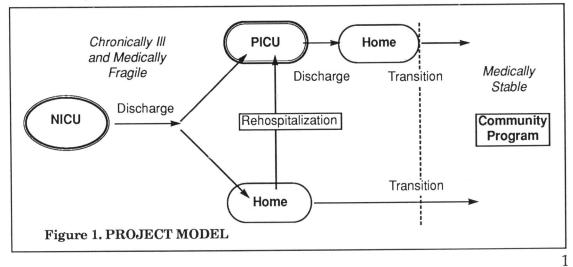

Figure 1. PROJECT MODEL

PROJECT COMPONENTS

NICU Component

Enrollment of CIII infants begins by identifying NICU babies who would be expected to have a prolonged initial NICU stay or would be at high risk for multiple rehospitalizations during their first two years because of their low birthweight, immaturity, and/or neonatal illness. Once identified, candidates are monitored until their health status suggests a good chance of immediate survival. At that time parents are approached with an explanation of the CIII Project and are invited to participate. An infant born at 25 weeks gestation is typically ready for enrollment in four or five weeks. At enrollment, a CIII staff member assumes the role of **case manager** for the family to coordinate project activities for the duration of the family's involvement in the CIII Project.

Upon acceptance into the Project, the CIII infants and their families receive a comprehensive intervention program delivered by professionals in the following disciplines:

- Special Education -- developmental recommendations based on behavioral observations of the infant
- Physical or Occupational Therapy -- a therapeutic program including positioning and handling techniques
- Nursing -- a carefully coordinated discharge plan
- Psychology -- consultation to the team regarding psychosocial issues of the family and parent-professional collaboration.

The CIII **special educator** conducts a structured behavioral observation of each infant with the *Naturalistic Observation of Newborn Behavior* format developed by Heidelise Als (Als, 1984). This observation is designed to identify the premature infant's response to environmental stimulation. Patterns of behavioral responses are identified and become the basis for developmental recommendations to the infant's caregivers in the NICU (Als, 1986). The special educator meets with the family to share recommendations and to assist parents in reading their infant's cues and in responding appropriately. Developmental recommendations are also written in the communication book provided to each family and posted at the infant's bedside.

The CIII **physical or occupational therapist** conducts a neurological examination using the *Neonatal Neurobehavioral Exam* (Morgan et al, 1988) and develops a program consisting of optimal positions and handling techniques to normalize muscle tone. These activities are communicated to the infant's caregivers in the same manner as the special educator's recommendations.

Home-Based Component

Because the CIII infant's health status typically precludes immediate enrollment into a community infant program, the family receives CIII home-based intervention services when the infant is discharged home. The family's CIII case manager continues to assume primary responsibility for working with the family to coordinate intervention services. Approximately two weeks after discharge, the case manager arranges a **family-focused interview** (Winton and Bailey, 1988). All family members are invited to attend. The CIII psychologist and the CIII case manager usually participate in the meeting. The planning session assists the family in defining a plan of action for caring for the special needs of the infant at home and determining other related family needs. This meeting may be led by the CIII psychologist or case manager in the family home.

During the infant's first eight weeks at home, the home visits are typically scheduled as follows:

- initial weekly visits from the CIII nurse,
- a visit by the family's CIII case manager during week one or two, and
- visits by the therapist and the special educator on alternate weeks once the infant has stabilized at home (typically at week three or four).

An infant who needs medical supports or whose health is particularly fragile receives ongoing visits by the CIII nurse. Once the child's health is stable, intervention consists primarily of visits from the special educator and physical/occupational therapist. The specialists usually visit on an alternate week basis.

Intervention is coordinated with the results of the infant's DEC follow up assessments at 4, 8, 12, 18, and 24 months of age. When clinic results indicate normal motor and cognitive development and when there is no outstanding family need, specialists' visits are scaled down and ongoing contact is maintained by the case manager. When DEC results indicate motor or cognitive delays, visits by the physical/occupational therapist or special educator are continued and sometimes increased.

Between months 18 and 24, consideration is given to phasing the infant from the CIII Project into appropriate community services as needed. These services may include local special education center-based programs, home-based programs, private therapy, and regular day care centers. Should a CIII infant be medically stable but have a significant handicap and demonstrate a need for extensive daily intervention services, transition into a center-based program may occur earlier.

If, on the other hand, the infant's medical status precludes discharge to the home or if the infant requires rehospitalization, the PICU Component is implemented.

PICU Component

Some infants will need hospitalization in the PICU either directly from the NICU or, after initial discharge, from the home. Infants in the NICU requiring prolonged hospitalization may be transferred to the PICU when it is considered inappropriate for them to remain in the nursery because of their size and age.

Nurseries, both intensive care and transitional, are directed primarily to meeting the needs of the neonate and the very young infant.

Chronically ill and medically fragile infants may be rehospitalized during their first 18 months for numerous reasons. Within the CIII population, infants with severe bronchopulmonary dysplasia (BPD) or feeding intolerance have most often required discharge to the PICU. The hospital stay for these infants ranges from 5 to 13 months.

Many premature infants, especially those with BPD, are particularly susceptible to upper respiratory infections. For these infants, a respiratory virus can result in pulmonary infection that requires aggressive medical treatment in the hospital. Another major reason for rehospitalization is feeding problems, including the short bowel syndrome, which causes difficulties with absorption of food. In addition, the failure-to-thrive infant who does not gain weight at home is often rehospitalized for extensive nutritional and feeding consultations. Finally, some infants require repeated surgery to correct congenital abnormalities of the cardiac, gastrointestinal, and/or urinary systems.

During a CIII infant's stay on the PICU, the case manager continues to work with the family to coordinate intervention services. The nurse assists the family in understanding any new medical procedures and their implications, especially in planning for the infant's discharge home. The CIII team offers emotional support to the family who may need it in learning new procedures such as tracheostomy management for an infant with BPD. Sometimes families are put in touch with others whose children have undergone similar procedures. Special education and physical/occupational therapy services are continued when the hospitalized infant is medically stable. Once again, developmental recommendations are prepared, posted at bedside, and shared with family and hospital staff.

PROJECT PHILOSOPHY

The CIII Project components were designed to meet the needs of chronically ill and medically fragile infants and their families. The following elements underlie each aspect of the program:

- a family-centered approach to intervention,
- a case manager role, and
- interdisciplinary developmental programming.

Family-Centered Intervention

In spite of the overall lack of rigorous research demonstrating the effectiveness of early intervention, parental involvement is the one aspect that has most clearly been demonstrated as an essential component in effective intervention (Shonkoff and Hauser-Cram, 1987). The parent's role as primary caregiver can be complicated by the specialized medical care required by the chronically ill infant during the first months of life. The CIII staff works to facilitate optimal bonding

4

and attachment between the infant and parent. The development of parental competence in managing their infant is emphasized. The staff initially offer suggestions for parental interaction and, as the child's medical condition stabilizes, the parental caregiving role is expanded.

Parents receive assistance in assuming the role of primary care providers. At the hospital, parents are encouraged to take a primary caregiving role whenever possible with diapering, feeding, and bathing. By participating in caregiving during the initial hospital stay, parents develop the skills necessary to care for the complex needs of their infant. As parents become more accustomed to providing this care, they are less anxious regarding the physical caregiving and can more easily focus on the infant's developmental needs.

Parents participate actively in decisions regarding the intervention services provided by the CIII Project which maintains a family-centered approach in all three components. Parental input regarding family strengths and needs are elicited, particularly during the family-focused meeting shortly after discharge. These perceptions along with specific developmental assessments of the infant are used to design the intervention program for the home-based component.

Parents can provide professionals with valuable information regarding the services received. Thus all parents are asked to provide regular feedback regarding the usefulness and effectiveness of the services and the sensitivity of the staff. This feedback is used by staff for appropriate modification of services. In addition, parents of chronically ill infants serve along with a group of professionals on an advisory board to the Project and provide formal feedback regarding CIII Project activities.

Role of the CIII Case Manager

The vast range of medical and developmental needs of chronically ill infants necessitates extensive coordination of services. As mentioned, each CIII family has a case manager to oversee coordination of services. Each member of the CIII intervention team becomes a case manager for an equal number of families.

When the need for long-term intervention is obvious at enrollment, the specialist who will provide major intervention assumes the role of case manager. For example, the CIII nurse typically becomes case manager for infants who have major physical anomalies requiring repeated surgeries or ongoing follow up by medical specialists. In cases in which no specific long-term handicap of the infant can be identified at enrollment, any CIII team member may become the case manager. The case manager assumes the responsibilities listed in Table 1.

Interdisciplinary Developmental Programming

The experiences of the CIII Project indicate that the therapeutic and developmental needs of chronically ill and at risk infants and their families

Table 1

THE RESPONSIBILITIES OF THE CASE MANAGER

NICU Component
Liaison with hospital staff
  primary nurses
  social workers
  neonatologists
Assist in discharge planning
Family support
  enroll families
  maintain ongoing communication
Child intervention
  attend weekly CIII staffing
  coordinate developmental recommendations

Home-Based Component
Liaison with medical and nursing personnel
  primary pediatrician
  specialty clinics
  visiting and home-care nurses
Family support
  assist in identifying family needs
  attend family-focused interview
  maintain regular contact
  assist in accessing services
Child intervention
  attend weekly CIII staffing
  coordinate developmental plan

PICU Component
Liaison with hospital staff
  primary nurses
  social workers
  pediatricians
Family support
  identify family needs
  maintain ongoing communication
Child intervention
  attend PICU Child Life Rounds
  coordinate developmental plan
Assist in discharge planning

change in emphasis during the first 24 months. Awareness of these changes may prepare interventionists to address the relevant needs.

Caregiving and Emotional Support

During the early months of the infant's life, the family needs considerable *caregiving information* and *general emotional support*. Early parental needs reflect the fact that the birth of a chronically ill or medically fragile infant is a source of major stress for a family. Thus, parents depend on knowledgeable and sympathetic professionals for support.

During the infant's hospital stay, a wide range of professionals provide parents with continuous information. The transition to home care after three to four months of involvement in intensive care can be experienced as a withdrawal of needed help unless ongoing support is available. The CIII nurse is particularly helpful in assisting parents in the transition to full caregiving for their infant. The nurse may provide information to help parents organize the home environment to make apnea monitors, oxygen supply tanks, and other supplies easily accessible. During initial home visits the CIII nurse reviews with the parents the operation of equipment, reading early stress signs, and the administration of medications.

Suggestions for establishing routine caregiving activities such as feeding, bathing, and sleeping are important to parents during the first several months of home care. While these same issues concern parents of healthy newborns, the medical history of chronically ill infants may complicate management routines. Each member of the CIII team contributes to the development of successful management practices. The nurse typically assists the family in promoting appropriate day and night sleeping cycles and feeding habits. The physical/occupational therapist assists with positioning and handling techniques to diminish irritability and promote feeding and mobility. The special educator assists in arranging the environment to provide appropriate stimulation and in suggesting activities that foster developmental progress. The psychologist suggests ways to enhance parent-child interactions.

Developmental Support

Parents become increasingly interested in their child's educational development in terms of intellectual and language skills around one year of age and continuing through 18 months. This is often the time when the infant is medically stable and begins showing signs of developmental "catch-up" in growth and abilities. Cognitive concepts (e.g., object permanence, imitation, understanding cause and effect) and language development are targeted for home activities at this time. Encouraging opportunities for cognitive activities and parent-child communication is important. The CIII special educator makes suggestions to enhance play interactions between the parents and their infant.

Intervention for optimal *motor development*, however, appears to be a consistent need throughout the first 18 months. The ongoing need for motor input over the first 18 months may stem from the fact that delayed motor development is common among chronically ill premature infants (Ellison, Browning and Horn, 1983). Developmental theorists consider the first 18 months of life to be the sensorimotor stage of development. Infants learn about themselves, their environment, and their interactions primarily through their motoric and sensory systems. Infants with motor delay may not be able to engage in activities necessary for optimal cognitive development. Motor input enables the infant to better engage in environmental experiences important for development.

While interdisciplinary programming is clearly warranted for the chronically ill infant during the first two years, CIII specialists sometimes alternate their home visiting schedules so that the changing needs of both the infant and family can be adequately addressed. This may mean frequent home visits by the nurse initially and by the special educator later as the infant becomes medically stable. In a few cases, families may not tolerate more than one visitor. In these cases, the transdisciplinary approach may be utilized; a primary interventionist integrates input from the various disciplines for the identified needs. The intervention specialists must be prepared to deal with their own disciplinary concerns as well as with a wide range of general and specific parental and developmental concerns.

ADAPTATION OF THE MODEL

Adapting the CIII model to another facility may involve utilizing other available disciplines and defining individual team roles to accommodate both the skills of individual team members and the needs of the families served. Although the disciplines represented on the CIII team include special education, physical and occupational therapy, nursing, and psychology, other disciplines could serve similar functions on the team. For example, a social worker could perform several of the functions of the CIII nurse, particularly identifying, accessing, and coordinating community services after discharge. A pediatric psychologist could serve some of the roles of the special educator, particularly in the NICU component.

The remainder of this guide describes the provision of services to chronically ill infants and their families in the three settings used in the CIII Project - NICU, home, and PICU. This guide is written for neonatal and pediatric caregivers as well as for staff at developmental centers who are interested in providing comprehensive services for chronically ill infants. It provides the basic information to design and implement a program that assures continuity in services for this group of vulnerable infants and their families.

2 INTERVENTION IN THE NEONATAL INTENSIVE CARE UNIT

INITIATING A DEVELOPMENTAL INTERVENTION PROGRAM: GAINING ADMINISTRATIVE SUPPORT

In order for an intervention program to succeed in a hospital setting, it must have wide support from the various administrative components of the medical and nursing units involved. Included among these would be:

- chief neonatologist,
- staff neonatologists,
- nursing coordinator,
- assistant nurse coordinators,
- staff nurses, and
- social service providers.

Developmental interventionists also need to identify the specific individuals who may be key to affecting changes in the unit by force of personality rather than particular administrative position.

The administrative organization of the NICU varies from facility to facility. For example, the administrative hierarchy at Georgetown University Hospital is presented in Figure 2. Neonatology is a division within the Department of Pediatrics with the Division Chief of Neonatology serving as Director of the Nurseries.

At Georgetown University, the Child Development Center is also a division within the Department of Pediatrics. If an intervention program for the NICU is to be developed by staff from another division within the hospital, any prior relationship between neonatology and that division may facilitate the new program. At Georgetown University, the Child Development Center has provided a NICU graduate follow-up clinic for many years. Thus, the Child Development Center and the Division of Neonatology had an already existing relationship. In addition, several collaborative developmental outcome studies had been pursued by the follow-up clinic staff and neonatologists. These prior collaborative efforts facilitated both the acceptance and implementation of a developmental program within the NICU.

When the developmental intervention is proposed from outside the hospital or from a division with little or no history of prior collaboration with neonatology staff, greater efforts may need to be made to gain the interest and support of the NICU administrative staff. In any case, developmental staff will need a carefully designed plan for garnering administrative support in order to assure that the developmental program is well received and effective. Elements of such a plan are described in this section.

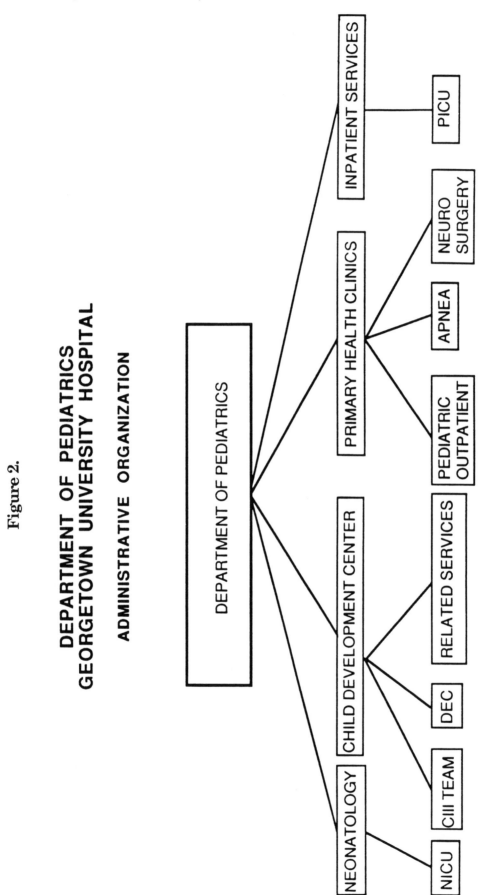

Figure 2.

DEPARTMENT OF PEDIATRICS
GEORGETOWN UNIVERSITY HOSPITAL

ADMINISTRATIVE ORGANIZATION

It is imperative to involve the chief neonatologist from the beginning. The objectives and procedures should be discussed with the neonatologist to assure his/her acceptance and understanding. In addition, developmental staff should attempt to elicit suggestions from the chief administrator regarding introducing the proposed program to other neonatology attending physicians. The chief neonatologist may wish to call a meeting and introduce the developmental program and staff to the attending physicians. Developmental staff will do well to have a carefully thought out agenda to clarify goals and components of the developmental program and to elicit potential concerns and suggestions for implementation. A slide presentation can be an effective method for introducing program goals and developmental staff to attending physicians.

It is sometimes possible to identify a particular ally among attending neonatologists who has a special interest in either developmental intervention or family issues. This person may play a key role in seeing that developmental services are accessed as the program is set in motion.

Because neonatologists need to focus on rapidly changing advances in neonatal medicine, some may not be as current about the literature on developmental techniques. Some physicians may be aware of the literature on overstimulation and have a negative impression of the role of intervention because they equate intervention with potentially harmful infant stimulation. Description of such studies as Als et al. (1986) and reviews by Bennett (1987) and Gorski et al. (1987) may help familiarize physicians with current efficacy studies of NICU intervention. Emphasis on the non-intrusive aspects of current intervention approaches may help alleviate some physicians' concerns about compromising very sick infants.

Providing physicians with up-to-date information on effective developmental program approaches may be done through several different strategies. One would be to make articles available at a division meeting or at journal club. Another approach would be to participate in a departmental grand rounds focused on developmental intervention in the nursery.

An area of intervention to emphasize in garnering physicians' support is that of developmental consultation to parents. Parents of NICU infants often become preoccupied with watching monitors of heart rate and oxygen saturation rates. They become very anxious about minor changes in these readings. Their preoccupation with the NICU technology may interfere with their ability to process more important information regarding their baby's status. It may even interfere with their ability to relate emotionally to the infant. Providing the parents with another framework by which to observe their baby's status and progress may improve both parent-infant and parent-physician relations.

Developmental interventionists in NICUs at teaching hospitals should also seek ways to inform residents about the developmental intervention. These individuals are actively involved in serving the medical needs of NICU infants and should be as involved as much as possible in promoting developmental intervention. Unfortunately, because of rotation and other scheduling problems, it is sometimes difficult to involve residents. However, if a mechanism can be found for introducing residents to the developmental program early in their rotation, it will usually be possible to identify those individuals specifically interested in promoting developmental awareness.

Nursing Administration and Staff

A meeting with the administrative nursing director for the nursery is another essential early step in implementing a developmental program in the NICU. This meeting can be designed to serve a two-fold purpose. First, the administrator can be introduced to the goals of the intervention as well as each of the intervention staff. In addition, intervention staff can be given a detailed description of the nurse staffing patterns. Nurse staffing patterns are often complex systems with varying levels of administrative coordination. For example, at Georgetown University Hospital, the nurseries have 38 beds with a rotating nursing staff of 90. A group of five Assistant Nurse Coordinators (ANCs) comprises the administrative level below the Nursing Coordinator. In addition, several neonatal nurse practitioners are responsible for maintaining the standards of care delivered to individual infants [Figure 3]. Developmental intervention teams must become familiar with the key nursing positions in order to determine the critical contacts to maintain support for the overall developmental intervention program as well as for programs for individual infants.

While making research literature available to the nursing coordinator and staff is beneficial, providing information on the pragmatic aspects of the intervention is especially important for the staff involved with direct care. Nurses who are already heavily burdened with medical caregiving responsibility need to know how they can incorporate developmental caregiving goals in a practical way. They need to know the benefits of what they are asked to do. In addition, if they are to have an incentive to pursue developmental goals, nurses must play an active role in formulating the intervention plan for infants under their care. Early meetings with administrative staff can be useful in formulating strategies for promoting the *facilitator role* of the nurses during their routine caregiving. A needs assessment in which nurses report their relative interest in areas of developmental information can be a helpful preliminary step for involving staff nurses.

Providing Preservice and Inservice Training to Nursing Staff

Once preliminary meetings with administrative nursing staff have been undertaken, the intervention team must develop and implement a nursery wide training plan for nursing staff. Optimally, inservice training sessions will need to be repeated for various shifts. This may mean sessions held at 8 am, 4 pm and 11 pm. However, the authors' experience indicated that inservice staff meetings held during the nurses regular shift were not effective in reaching the majority of the 90 nurses staffing the unit. Often nurses are unable to attend because of tight staffing

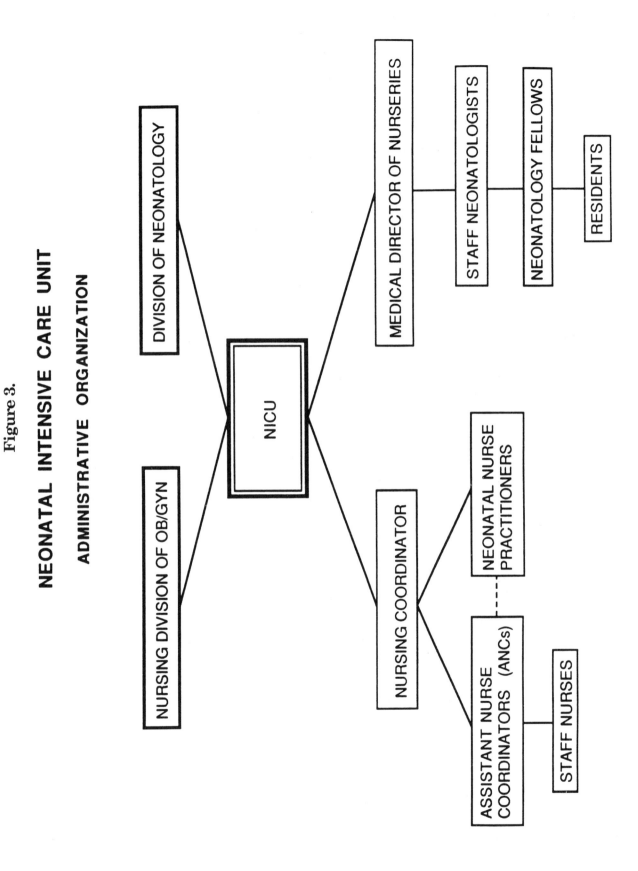

Figure 3.

NEONATAL INTENSIVE CARE UNIT

ADMINISTRATIVE ORGANIZATION

or unexpected crises on the unit. A short term solution may be to introduce the intervention program and team members through the use of a notebook. A pictorial description in a photo album can be left in the nurses' lounge where nurses check off their names after they review the notebook and respond to a *needs assessment* made available with the notebook. The needs assessment can consist of a checklist of developmental topics for future training sessions. Topics that might be listed include: positioning techniques, developmental outcome for high risk infants, normal neonatal development. The nurses indicate their interest level for each item. These forms actively involve nurses in the developmental program and serve as a guide for planning future information sharing sessions.

Providing inservice training regarding developmental intervention to at least a core of nurses remains an essential task of the developmental team if intervention is going to be carried out throughout the infant's stay in the NICU. In some hospitals a few nurses have been involved with developmental intervention through nursing conferences. At Georgetown University Hospital, the nurses themselves formed a developmental committee as a result of their participation in a seminar on the impact of the NICU environment on the developing premie. As a result, a number of the NICU nurses had begun to meet to discuss how adaptations could be made in the Georgetown nurseries to promote infant development. While the developmental committee was organized by the nurses, it also had participation from neonatology, nursing administration, social work, and the special educator from the Child Development Center.

The committee developed the following set of objectives:
- To educate the NICU staff to the psychosocial and neuromotor needs of premature and chronically ill infants.
- To assist NICU staff in improving handling techniques and positioning with the infants.
- To assist NICU staff in helping parents read behavioral signs of their infants.
- To assist NICU staff in making adaptations to the NICU environment to reduce unnecessary intrusions on the infant.

The committee attempted to communicate these goals to the wider staff. Several one hour inservice sessions were scheduled and reading material was provided in the nurses' lounge and at the nurses' station.

Since most NICUs do not have an organized developmental committee, the developmental team is left to determine how developmental information can be shared with the majority of staff. Communicating on a one-to-one basis with nurses is important but is inefficient, especially in the beginning of a new program. A more effective method is to gather a substantial percentage of the staff for a one or two day developmental conference.

Any of a number of specific plans can be used for developmental conferences. A two day session can be undertaken if administrators are willing to pay nurses for attending both days. Continuing education units can also be negotiated for the sessions. The session can then be repeated for another segment of the nurses. In this way a substantial portion of the staff nurses receive information about developmental intervention. If a two day session is a larger committment than the hospital is ready to make, then a one day or even a partial day can be set aside to provide staff release time to learn about developmental intervention in the NICU. Optimally, the session will be repeated so that at least 50 percent of the staff will receive the information and, hopefully, be ready to work with the developmental team in implementing a comprehensive program for the infants and their families.

In whatever way possible, a developmental team about to embark on providing intervention in the NICU will need a vehicle to communicate with a substantial portion of the NICU nurses. Each institution will have to determine the most effective way to provide this communication.

As the developmental intervention program is implemented in the NICU, developmental staff will also need to consider the most effective way to provide information on developmental intervention to neonatal nurses joining the unit. Once again, it is essential to work with administrative staff in determining a mechanism for incorporating developmental training into the regular orientation program. This may mean that developmental specialists will be asked to provide lectures or demonstrations during each new orientation program. The investment of time will be well worth the effort.

Timing of the Intervention

Once developmental intervention has been approved by the managers of the NICU, it is essential that the physicians be kept informed and approve plans to intervene with a particular infant and his/her family. Because final responsibility for the welfare of the infant lies with that physician, he or she must be aware and in support of non-medical plans for the infant as well.

Information from the physician may play an important role in the timing of the intervention with the infant and his family. For the very sick infant, concern will necessarily be focused on the acute medical crisis. In addition, very early in the NICU stay, the family may be overwhelmed by the crisis and environment such that input from yet another professional may be too much for them to process. The neonatologist in conjunction with nursing and social service staff usually is able to determine when additional input is appropriate.

On the other hand, for some families, work with the developmental specialist may provide an alternative way for them to relate to their baby. Those families who are excessively preoccupied with minor medical fluctuations put great stress on themselves and the nursery staff. Preoccupation with the medical equipment sometimes results when parents are looking for ways to do something for their baby. Providing a developmental focus may help them see themselves actively contributing to their infant's well being.

The authors have found that the developmental team usually does not initiate work directly with the family until the infant is several weeks old. For very small premature infants or others with major medical complications, it usually requires a few weeks before even short term survival can be predicted. It seems appropriate for developmental staff not to approach parents earlier than this point to discuss programming that would occur after discharge.

Participation in Family Service Rounds

Many NICU's have a weekly staff meeting called **Family Rounds** or **Social Service Rounds**. The meeting is attended by those staff members having contact with the family (usually the neonatologist, primary nurse and social worker). During these Rounds, information on family functioning and needs is discussed. Communication problems are identified and strategies are developed to facilitate improved communication with family members. Other stresses requiring services are identified, and ways to foster parent-infant attachment are developed.

Participation of a developmental team member in these Rounds may be useful in fulfilling the following:

1. Identifying infants appropriate for intervention,
2. Securing approval and support from the neonatologist to provide intervention to a particular infant, and
3. Providing input about family issues identified by developmental staff working with an infant already receiving intervention.

Developmental team members can often contribute at Rounds based on their extensive experience with families of at risk and handicapped children. Their presence also provides visibility for the intervention project to the administrative staff. Attendance at Rounds is also useful in keeping the attending staff informed of the status of developmental intervention for individual infants and in encouraging nursery staff to make referrals of infants and families who they feel would benefit from developmental intervention.

Ongoing Communication with Nursing Staff

Consistent communication between developmental specialists and nursing caregivers concerning the needs of infants is an essential component of developmental intervention in the NICU. Each infant's nurses play a critical role in carrying over developmental intervention to the infant and family. Developmental team members' communications must, therefore, be designed to facilitate the nursing staff's role in the delivery of intervention. Unfortunately, however, the nursing staff in NICUs may be very large and experience substantial yearly turnover. This makes the task of ongoing communication difficult.

In some settings a primary care nurse system is used. In this case, one nurse is assigned to regular caregiving for a particular infant and may be considered the primary liaison for the family. In other NICUs, primary nurses are not assigned to individual infants because of nursery rotation schedules, etc. However, a primary team of nurses may exist with several nurses providing most of the care for the infant during the week. In some cases a nurse will take an interest in a particular baby, especially the chronic baby, and request frequent assignment to that infant. In each case, the appropriate nurse or nurses need to be identified as the primary contact(s) for the developmental team.

In situations where a primary contact nurse is identified, the team members can communicate directly with that nurse in explaining developmental objectives. When no particular nurse is considered primary, the team will need to discuss objectives with a number of the nurses providing care for the infant. In some cases it may be helpful to post a note requesting interested nurses to meet with the developmental team to discuss an individual infant's developmental concerns. Posting developmental recommendations on the isolette can also facilitate communication especially when many nurses are taking care of an individual baby during the course of each week. Maintaining communication with the infant's caregivers remains a considerable challenge for developmental teams and usually necessitates a variety of creative approaches.

Providing Staff Information on Outcome

While developmental teams are usually in the position of requesting cooperation from nursing staff, teams may provide a real service to NICU staff by providing them with information on later development of the infants they care for. Physicians and nurses are often very gratified when they are able to see older infants they cared for previously in the NICU. Developmental teams who provide intervention to infants after discharge from the NICU are in the position of providing nursery staff with information on developmental outcome.

If the same developmental intervention team is involved with regular developmental clinic follow-up visits, families may be encouraged to return for a brief visit to the NICU to "show off" their infants. When possible, schedules of infants coming for evaluation during the week can be provided to the NICU staff so that nurses who are available can stop by the clinic and say hello to the family. Photographs of individual infants can be taken either at clinic visits or during home visits and then circulated in the NICU for staff to see. A more formal effort may include framing a collection of photographs of infants several months to a year after discharge. Such a collection is typically cherished by the NICU staff and displayed in a prominant place. These fairly simple efforts provide positive reinforcement for the staff's hard work in the NICU and promote greater collaboration between nursery staff and the developmental team.

Summary

Implementation of the NICU intervention program in the nursery requires garnering support of medical and nursing administrative staff before the program begins. Mutual support and respect for each other's roles are essential if the program is to be effective. Maintaining regular communication among the multiple care providers and the developmental team requires a variety of strategies but is important because it results in better support for the family and more effective intervention for the infant.

SPECIAL EDUCATION IN THE NICU

Twenty years ago, special educators worked almost exclusively with the school age population within traditional educational systems. The movement toward remedial education began in the late 1960's with concern about socially disadvantaged populations. In more recent years concern has focused on handicapped young children. Legislative impetus for this concern came in 1975 when Public Law 94-142 was enacted. This Education for All Handicapped Children Act, while directed primarily at the school age population, also provided incentive monies to states for early intervention services for children with special needs between the ages of three and five. A number of states also initiated early intervention programs for handicapped infants from birth through two years of age.

Programs focusing on handicapped and at-risk infants have received further impetus through the passage of Public Law 99-457. These amendments enacted in 1986 directed states to begin a five-year planning process to implement intervention services to all developmentally delayed infants from birth through two years of age.

The Role of Special Education in the NICU

Health, education and social service agencies are working together in each state to develop a comprehensive service delivery system that meets the needs of these special infants and their families. As states develop programs to meet the needs of chronically ill infants, special educators will become increasingly involved with very young, developmentally delayed and at risk infants. As this happens, more educators will work within the hospital.

Academic departments of universities are presently developing programs or adopting curricula to prepare special education personnel to meet the needs of handicapped infants and their families. Hopefully these programs will address the development of skills that will be needed by special educators working with chronically ill and medically fragile infants and their families in the NICU. Special educators working in the NICU may need to assume a variety of the roles within hospitals including the roles of infant specialist, facilitator/consultant, parent educator, program developer, and advocate (Geik et al., 1982).

The special educator must function as **an infant specialist** with skills in identifying the *physical and behavioral responses* of the chronically ill infant. In the NICU, the specialist must have a firm grasp of the behavior of the normal full-term infant as well as the at risk neonate. In addition, the specialist needs information and skills in *intervention strategies* with both the ill full-term infant and the premature infant. Behavioral responses and intervention strategies differ for infants at various stages. For example, the acutely ill infant and the stable, growing premie each have different needs. The infant specialist must be prepared to work with infants at each of these stages.

The NICU arena demands that a special educator function as a **facilitator** and **consultant** with skills to observe, understand, and communicate about the infant's behavioral responses to the environment. Because of the medical instability and fragility of hospitalized infants, the special educator will often find it necessary to intervene with the infant through suggestions to staff and parents rather than in a "hands on" capacity. The specialist interprets the infant's behaviors and recommends developmental interventions which are then provided, for the greater part, through the primary nursing and medical caregivers in the NICU. Unfortunately, teacher preparation programs often fail to emphasize skills in working with adults. The special educator who knows how to work with both infants and adults is better prepared to work effectively in the NICU.

The special educator working in the NICU will also need to function in the **parent educator role**. The special educator in the NICU plays an important role in helping parents understand their infant's sometimes unexpected and immature behavioral responses. In addition, the special educator can help prepare parents to interact successfully with the infant by assisting parents in noticing the infant's subtle behavioral cues.

A final area in which the NICU special educator must function is that of **program developer** and **advocate**. Because developmental intervention in the NICU is in its formative stages, the special educator will need to keep abreast of research findings and work to apply these findings to develop more effective intervention strategies. In addition, the special educator will need to advocate for developmental intervention in NICU environments which up to now, have focused primarily on medical interventions. While recognizing the critical need for ongoing and often intrusive medical treatment, the special educator in the NICU will need to advocate for the ongoing developmental needs of both the infant and the parents. As a fairly new hospital team member, the special educator must be able to identify those strategies which will result in effective advocacy.

NICU Infants Receiving Intervention from the Special Educator

Infants in special care nurseries are a particularly heterogenous group. Typically, nurseries are divided into two sections to address two very different sets of needs within the total population of special care infants:

- *Neonatal Intensive Care Unit*: infants who are medically unstable and typically require mechanical ventilation, and
- *Neonatal Intermediate Care Unit (Transition or Step Down Nurseries)*: infants who have stabilized and may no longer require mechanical ventilation, but who often require supplemental oxygen and/or have not yet met discharge weight criterion.

The first developmental task of preterm infants is to adapt to extrauterine life despite the fact that their bodies have not developed completely. Medical problems may arise as the premature infant fails physiologically to accommodate to the demands of extrauterine life or as medical interventions, given to perform the functions for which premies are not ready (e.g., feeding, breathing, thermal regulation) produce further, if unavoidable, harm.

Special groups of infants in the intensive care and intermediate nurseries who benefit from developmental intervention include:

- Premature infants who because of *extreme immaturity* and/or low birth weight are in need of extended hospital stay.
- The infant who develops *BPD* and whose respiratory system continues to be compromised. These infants, even after 35 weeks gestational age, are often extremely irritable and difficult to console. They typically have poor weight gain and usually have a long stay in the transitional nursery before discharge home.
- Premature and full-term infants with *specific medical problems* such as short bowel syndrome requiring long-term hospital medical treatment. These infants also share prolonged stays in the transitional nursery. They sometimes outgrow the nursery and are transferred to the pediatric units when they are six or seven months old.
- Premature and full-term infants born with *multiple congenital anomalies* requiring repeated surgeries before and after discharge to home.
- Infants with *central nervous system insult* that damages autonomic functions such as breathing, feeding and handling secretions.

The Nature of Intervention

As stated earlier, the NICU environment typically provides excessive and inappropriate patterns of stimulation to premature infants. The special educator can be helpful in sensitizing NICU staff to the presence of this stimulation and to strategies for reducing it. In addition, the special educator's roles in the NICU is to observe the individual infant's behavioral responses in order to identify appropriate developmental interventions. These areas are discussed briefly below.

Improving the NICU Environment

An important portion of the special educator's emphasis is on working through NICU staff to improve the overall NICU environment so that all infants and their families benefit. A major role consists of assisting staff in reducing excess stimulation from three general sources: **noise, light, and activity.**

In order to be effective in improving the NICU environment, the special educator will need to provide information on the potential effects of stimulation occurring in the NICU. In addition, the special educator must be viewed as a member of the nursery team who contributes to creative problem solving. The special educator works collaboratively with nursery staff during staff development sessions and through one-to-one interactions. The more informed the NICU staff is regarding the deleterious effects of stimuli on the infants, the more motivated they will be to work together to reduce excess stimulation.

Specific strategies for reducing excess stimulation from noise, light and activity within the NICU environment are presented in Table 2.

Table 2

STRATEGIES FOR REDUCING EXCESS NOISE

- Gently lower the head on the isolette mattress tray.
- Close portholes and isolette cabinets quietly.
- Set feeding bottles in places other than the top of isolettes.
- Eliminate finger tapping on isolettes.
- Move loud machinery such as computer printers out of the NICU.
- Encourage staff to silence alarms as soon as possible and to silence the ventilator alarm prior to suctioning.
- Discontinue the audible heart rate beeps.
- Reduce talking over the isolette or across rooms.
- Eliminate radios or reduce their use to designated periods and confine music to calm, soothing music.

STRATEGIES FOR REDUCING BRIGHT LIGHTING

- Cover isolettes with blankets to reduce the amount of bright light that filters into individual isolettes.
- Dim the lights on a regular schedule, especially in transitional units, to reduce light levels as well as to promote normal day-night cycles.
- Cover infant's eyes with patches during procedures with the heat and bilirubin lamps and shield infants in adjoining isolettes.

STRATEGIES FOR REDUCING EXCESS ACTIVITY

- Move less acute infants to a quieter area.
- Establish quiet times in the nursery when activity as well as light and noise are reduced.

Assessment for Programming for Individual Infants

Another role that the special educator plays is that of facilitating developmentally appropriate interventions for individual infants. Individual intervention is facilitated by the use of assessment measures to determine the infant's response to the environment. Both the Als *Naturalistic Observation of*

Newborn Behavior and the *Brazelton Neonatal Behavioral Assessment Scale (BNBAS)* can be used in intervention in the NICU.

The *Naturalistic Observation of Newborn Behavior* was developed by Als (1984) as a tool to identify behavioral responses of premature infants. The special educator conducts an observation of each enrolled premature infant several times during their NICU stay. Signs of infant stress and self regulation are noted. Observations are made approximately ten minutes prior to handling by a nurse, parent, or other person; during handling; and approximately ten minutes after handling. Observations are recorded in two-minute intervals during which all behaviors and observable changes of the infant are noted. Examples of observed behavioral responses are presented in Table 3.

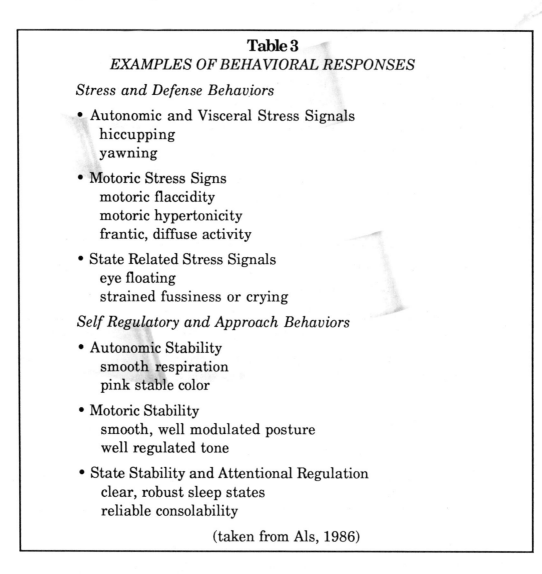

Table 3

EXAMPLES OF BEHAVIORAL RESPONSES

Stress and Defense Behaviors

• Autonomic and Visceral Stress Signals
  hiccupping
  yawning

• Motoric Stress Signs
  motoric flaccidity
  motoric hypertonicity
  frantic, diffuse activity

• State Related Stress Signals
  eye floating
  strained fussiness or crying

Self Regulatory and Approach Behaviors

• Autonomic Stability
  smooth respiration
  pink stable color

• Motoric Stability
  smooth, well modulated posture
  well regulated tone

• State Stability and Attentional Regulation
  clear, robust sleep states
  reliable consolability

(taken from Als, 1986)

The observations reveal the infant's patterns of responses to stimulation. The special educator identifies these patterns and provides recommendations to improve the infant's functioning either by reducing stress or enhancing self-regulatory behaviors.

A second tool used by the special educator is the *Brazelton Neonatal Behavioral Assessment Scale*. The BNBAS (Brazelton, 1984) is a behavioral and psychological exam for the infant between 37 and 44 weeks gestation who does not need ventilator support and is on room air. The BNBAS provides the special educator with the opportunity to interact with the older infant in the NICU in order to identify individual behavioral responses of the infant.

The seven functional response patterns that are assessed include: *habituation, orientation, motor, range of state, regulation of state, autonomic regulation, and reflexes.* The assessment of the infant usually takes about 30 minutes and involves approximately 30 different tasks or maneuvers.

The special educator may find it useful to administer the BNBAS to infants as they reach their expected date of delivery. Having been standardized on full-term infants, the BNBAS has only limited value for use with premies prior to 37 week gestation. Results of the infant's functioning in each of the seven areas can be shared with parents and NICU staff. Recommendations regarding the adjustment of auditory and/or visual stimulation can be made according to these results. For example, simple tracking activities can be recommended for an infant who shows readiness by visually focusing on an object. Other recommendations regarding the infant's response patterns can also be formulated and shared. Several major areas regarding the environment and direct caregiving techniques can be highlighted.

Since recommendations from both the *Naturalistic Observation of Newborn Behavior* and the *BNBAS* often cluster around general environmental changes and direct caregiving techniques, each of these areas are discussed in detail.

General Environmental Changes

One area that may be targeted for recommendations is the location of the infant's crib or isolette. Observation of an infant may reveal particular sensitivity to environmental noises. These infants will benefit from the removal of noise-producing items such as a radio or trash container. Moving the infant's crib or isolette to a quieter area of the nursery away from higher activity and noise levels may enhance the infant's functioning. Likewise, other infants may exhibit stress reactions to lights in the environment and may benefit from having the crib or isolette covered with blankets to reduce light levels.

A second more proximal environmental concern may involve the infant's bedding and clothing. Provision of a water mattress or tight nesting with blanket rolls may be suggested to assist restfulness or flexion. In addition, a hat, clothing, or swaddling blanket may be recommended to provide an individual infant with needed boundaries to facilitate sleep. These recommendations are particularly beneficial for infants who demonstrate frequent arching and other postural extension or high levels of irritability.

Observation of individual premies may suggest readiness for opportunities to promote self-regulatory behaviors. In these cases, it would be recommended that the premie be provided with opportunities to grasp onto fingers or finger rolls during manipulations or to suck a pacifier during and between feedings.

Finally, identification of positions that result in the infant's optimal functioning as well as supports to help maintain optimal positions are recommendations that may be particularly helpful for certain infants in the NICU.

Caregiving Techniques

Careful timing and sequencing of caregiving routines can help facilitate an infant's development. Assisting caregivers, nurses and parents in identifying the infant's behavioral responses is the first step in helping them adjust caregiving to meet the individual infant's needs.

A number of specific strategies may be recommended to modify caregiving according to individual infant's developmental needs. One strategy includes pausing at the first signs of stress to allow the infant to recuperate. Positioning the infant with shoulder and truncal support and foot bracing may be suggested for the infant who shows strong stress reactions to caregiving. Maintaining an infant in prone or sidelying during procedures may also be recommended especially for the unstable infant who does not tolerate the supine position. Clustering of intrusive procedures so they are not dispersed over a long period of time may also help an infant who sustains a strong stress reaction to such caregiving.

To enhance successful feeding, it may be useful to recommend that feedings be scheduled according to the infant's natural sleep cycle. This can help avoid interruption of deep sleep on the one hand, and eliminate periods of exhaustive crying before feeding, on the other hand. This recommendation should be made only in consultation with the medical and nursing staff to assure that the infant continues to receive adequate nutrition. When an infant is gavage fed, feeding inside a visually shielded isolette can help to reduce light levels for the infant who is particularly sensitive to visual stimulation. When an infant is breast- or bottle-fed, conducting feeding in a quiet corner behind a screen or in the parent room can be a useful strategy to decrease the stress and fatigue that is often a part of feeding for the premature infant.

The sample recommendations described here represent some of the major areas of concern identified through the use of the *Naturalistic Observation of Newborn Behavior*. After the observation and developmental recommendations are formulated, a descriptive report is written. These recommendations are shared with the infant's nurse and a discussion of special considerations and any necessary clarification is provided. Specific recommendations are posted on the infant's isolette or bed and are shared with the parents.

This approach to identifying intervention strategies within the NICU is observational and eliminates additional handling of the infant by the special educator. Chronically ill infants often receive extensive handling for necessary intrusive medical procedures even though these procedures may be extremely taxing to the infant. Further handling, even for developmental purposes, may be detrimental and should be minimized whenever possible. *The Naturalistic Observation of Newborn Behavior* allows the observer to gather extensive behavioral information on each infant without extra handling.

This description of the special educator's role in identifying and implementing developmental recommendations for individual infants highlights the facilitative nature of this role. The special educator must work through the infant's regular caregivers, particularly the nursing staff and the parents, if developmental recommendations are to be effective.

Developmental Recommendations and Parents

Supporting the role of parents as caregivers to their infant is important throughout the infant's stay in the NICU. Though their physical caregiving may be limited during the infant's initial acute state, parents can receive results of developmental observations to help them identify their infant's behavioral responses to the environment. This is particularly important in the early stages as the parents are adjusting to the premature birth and beginning the process of bonding.

Developmental recommendations related to caregiving procedures, in particular, provide parents with a better understanding of their baby and his or her needs and often provide specific ways they can contribute to their infant's progress. Involvement of this nature fosters parental competence.

Since it may be difficult to meet frequently with parents of infants in the NICU because of evening or weekend visits by parents, the special educator needs to make special efforts to maintain ongoing contact with the family. This contact may be made directly by phone or indirectly through a case manager. A communication book provided to each family at the time of enrollment can be used to facilitate ongoing communication with parents. It can be kept at the infant's bed for developmental staff and parents to read and write in. Phone contacts can also be made to respond to questions noted by parents in the book.

No matter what vehicle is used to assure communication with parents, the special educator plays a crucial role in helping parents get to know their special infant very early in the infant's life. Pointing out their infant's special behavioral responses can be invaluable for parents as they learn to parent their premature infant.

Developmental Intervention and the NICU Staff

The facilitative model of intervention described above is effective because it respects the nursing and medical expertise of NICU staff and recognizes them as the infant's primary interveners. Developmental recommendations derived from observations are discussed with nursing staff and modified by their input when appropriate. During these discussions, nursing staff become familiar with the developmental interventions and adapt them when appropriate. As a result, nursing staff are more prepared and motivated to carry out recommendations in their day-to-day caregiving. Thus, the infant receives an intervention program that is provided within the context of ongoing caregiving. This facilitative model is in contrast to the expert model in which an outside professional presents an intervention program designed without input from the NICU staff.

Extensive sharing of both general developmental information and highly individualized recommendations occurs on a one-to-one basis between the special educator and nursing staff. Nevertheless, the special educator should recognize the importance of participating in formal inservice training for NICU staff. Sharing information regarding developmental concerns with groups of staff is a part of educating NICU staff regarding the developmental needs of the infants they serve, as well as sensitizing them to the developmental implications of all aspects of their caregiving.

PHYSICAL/OCCUPATIONAL THERAPY IN THE NICU

The last ten years have given rise to a proliferation of infant intervention programs providing physical and occupational therapy to at risk and handicapped children. Additionally, increasing numbers of therapists are working in NICUs. Because of the considerable overlap in the roles of physical and occupational therapists in the NICU, this section will be applicable to the professional in either occupational or physical therapy who has had specialized training in pediatric therapy.

The purpose of this section is to provide the pediatric (physical or occupational) therapist with the background information needed to initiate a therapeutic program in the NICU. The following discussion includes competencies needed by the therapists initiating treatment in the NICU, as well as assessment and intervention strategies.

Competencies of Physical/Occupational Therapists Providing Services in the NICU

Because of the vast array of factors which place an infant at risk for developmental sequelae, it is important that a therapist be knowledgeable in recent neonatal and developmental literature. This knowledge will be invaluable in helping the therapist formulate a treatment philosophy and appropriate intervention strategies. Being a member of an interdisciplinary team providing developmental services is extremely helpful and is recommended especially in the initial phases of program development in the NICU.

The Section on Pediatrics of the American Physical Therapy Association (Scull and Dietz, 1988) has developed *Competencies for Physical Therapists* working in intensive care nurseries. This document includes a range of competencies needed for:

- conducting a comprehensive neurobehavioral exam,
- designing and modifying a treatment plan, and
- consulting to the various team members and the family.

It has also been suggested (Campbell, 1986) that a preceptorship with a therapist experienced in working with infants in the NICU facilitates the development of competencies of an individual therapist.

Neuromotor Differences, Full-term vs Preterm

Because many of the infants appropriate for therapeutic intervention are preterm infants, it is important to review some of the differences between them and full-term babies and outline the neuromotor findings seen in the infant who is at risk for neuromotor dysfunction.

Babies born *full-term* (38-42 weeks) are typically able to interpret and integrate sensory information in a meaningful way. They are alert to and focus on a visual or auditory stimuli quickly and are able to sustain attention to a bright stimulus. During their first weeks, they display an increase in flexion of the extremities and a midline orientation.

The *preterm* baby, on the other hand, is not as well organized as the full-term. Sweeney (1985), a pediatric physical therapist, has described three high risk profiles of preterm or vulnerable infants. The **hypertonic profile** includes those infants who tend to be irritable and have a low tolerance for physical handling. Their movements tend to be disorganized and tremulous. There is poor midline orientation of the extremities and limited anti-gravity movement into flexion which results in extensor posturing. Decreased mobility in the oral musculature contributes to feeding difficulties.

A baby who displays a **hypotonic profile** is difficult to arouse, and has a tendency to mold very easily when held. To compensate for the low muscle tone, the baby will push his body into extension to stabilize, especially at the shoulders and hips. The hypotonic baby may also have feeding difficulties due to fatigue, a weak suck, and poor coordination of the suck-swallow mechanism.

These two profiles (the hypertonic and hypotonic profiles) describe the extreme patterns of movement seen in the preterm infant.

The typical **premie profile** includes hypotonia combined with a tendency to "fix" or push against the surface when placed in positions necessitating anti-gravity movement. This contributes to the common postural profile seen in the premature infant. This profile includes the following components:

- hyperextension of the neck,
- elevated and retracted shoulders,
- decreased midline arm movement,
- an excessively extended trunk,
- an immobile pelvis,
- infrequent anti-gravity movement of the lower extremities, and
- weight bearing on toes when held in standing.

This premie profile can interfere with the infant's development and, as a result, become problematic. Aspects of this profile typically become the focus of therapeutic intervention. Figure 4 outlines the three profiles described above.

Figure 4
HIGH RISK PROFILES

Hypertonic Profile	**Hypotonic Profile**
Irritable	Difficult to arouse
Low tolerance to handling	Molds very easily
Disorganized movements	Fixates at shoulders and hips
Extensor posturing	Weak suck
Decreased mobility of oral musculature	Poor coordination of suck-swallow mechanism

Premie Profile

Hypotonia and decreased anti-gravity movement
Postural profile including:
 hyperextension of the neck
 elevated and retracted shoulders
 decreased midline arm movements
 excessively extended trunk
 immobile pelvis
 weight bearing on toes when held in standing

Premie Profile

Assessment

As in other specialty areas of physical and occupational therapy, proper assessment of each baby is an essential first step in developing an effective intervention program. A thorough neurobehavioral assessment will include the following:

- neuromuscular maturation,
- motoric functioning,
- musculoskeletal abnormalities,
- oral motor functioning, and
- neurobehavioral response to handling.

Because of the medical fragility of the infant, it may be necessary to perform the evaluation over several visits. The baby may be unable to tolerate the amount of interaction necessary to gain all needed information in one visit.

There are many assessment tools available to the therapist. Table 4 highlights some of the more common ones currently in use.

Table 4
NEUROMOTOR ASSESSMENTS

Clinical Assessment of Gestational Age in the Newborn Infant.
(Dubowitz et al, 1970)

Neurological Examination of the Full Term Infant. (Prechtl, 1977)

Neonatal Behavioral Assessment Scale. (Brazelton, 1984)

Neurological Assessment of the Preterm and Full Term Newborn
Infant. (Dubowitz & Dubowitz, 1981)

Neonatal Neurobehavioral Examination. (Morgan et al, 1988)

Neurological Evaluation of the Maturity of Newborn Infants.
(Amiel-Tison, 1968)

Movement Assessment of Infants. (Chandler et al, 1980)

Test of Motor and Neurological Functions. (DeGangi et al, 1983)

Subtest of Qualitative Movement Findings.(Valvano & DeGangi, 1986).

The CIII Project therapist uses the *Neonatal Neurobehavioral Examination (NNE)* because of its simplicity and its brevity. The *NNE* (Morgan, et al, 1988) includes the range of items covered in many of the other neurobehavioral evaluations. The assessment takes approximately 10 to 15 minutes for the experienced therapist to complete. The *NNE* complements the Als *Naturalistic Observation of Newborn Behavior* and the *Brazelton Neonatal Behavioral Assessment Scale* which can be used by the special educator. The *NNE* provides information regarding reflex development, postural responses, muscle tone, and response to handling. This gives the therapist the information needed to formulate a therapeutic plan. The results are evaluated with consideration for the degree of prematurity.

Along with performing the formal assessment using the *NNE*, the therapist assesses the *quality* of the infant's movement patterns and resting posture. Qualitative findings include the effect of muscle tone variations on movement, and the ability to hold a position. This is essential information for developing an appropriate treatment plan.

The therapist also evaluates *oral motor control* during feeding. It is important to evaluate both the oral motor mechanism and the feeding situation to determine intervention needs. The oral mechanisms assessed by the therapist include oral reflexes, tongue mobility, coordination of sucking and swallowing and facial musculature balance. Situational issues addressed by the therapist include the feeding position and whether the baby is fed orally or by gavage. When introducing the bottle it is also necessary to assess the nipple chosen and energy expended, especially in the infant with respiratory problems.

In conducting an evaluation and in interpreting the results, the therapist must consider many factors. The degree of prematurity can affect the infant's behavior. Hypotonia and weak reflex development is normal for an early preterm baby in their first weeks of life. Evaluation findings during that period should reflect this fact. However, if a baby compensates for this hypotonia with hyperextension of the neck and retraction of the shoulders this will interfere with attempts to bring hands to midline, and should be noted as significant. Assessing the qualitative differences helps the therapist differentiate between "normal" preterm behavior and abnormal development. Other factors to consider include the amount or type of medication taken by the infant, the baby's fatigue level, and stimulation from the environment.

Intervention

Therapeutic intervention in the NICU is based on the results of a number of studies which have evaluated the effects of sensorimotor intervention on the preterm infant (Rose, et al. 1980; Campbell, 1983). Effective treatment plans are designed and implemented based on the perspective that the NICU environment exposes vulnerable infants to disjunctive patterns of stimulation. The five major goals of the therapeutic intervention include:

1. Normalizing muscle tone,
2. Minimizing postural disorganization,
3. Minimizing contractures and deformity,
4. Facilitating normal patterns of movement, and
5. Promoting appropriate feeding behavior.

The treatment plan developed for the infant in the NICU must be tailored to the individual infant's needs and tolerance level. The plan should be designed with consideration for any risk to the individual infant. Specific areas of concern include potential for:

- respiratory compromise during movements,
- aspiration during feeding,

• skin breakdown during positioning, taping, or splinting, and

• fracture or dislocation during movement of joints limited in range of motion.

It is of utmost importance that the therapist also be aware of physiologic stress signs. **Stress signs** include color changes, changes in breathing patterns, behavioral signs such as yawns, sneezing, gaze aversion, and hiccups, motor signs such as trunk arching, finger splaying, saluting, and stiffening of the extremities. At the onset of stress signs the therapist should respond by reducing stimulation to allow the infant to recuperate before continuing.

Although there are many strategies that can be integrated into a therapy program, concentrated efforts can be focused on two major categories: *positioning* and *sensorimotor activities*.

Positioning

Proper positioning which is integrated into the infant's daily routine can greatly affect the muscular imbalance often seen in the preterm infant. When placed in the supine position, the hypotonic baby often "fixes" against gravity contributing to the typical premie posture. Prone and sidelying, on the other hand, are the positions of choice as they enhance flexion and counteract shoulder retraction and neck hyperextension.

Proper positioning will help to counteract the premie posture and promote flexion and a midline orientation. The creative use of blankets, diaper, and/or towel rolls in prone, sidelying, and supine with head support can help to reach the objective of increased flexion. The flexed position is helpful in decreasing disorganized movements and facilitating the desirable hand to mouth behavior and midline orientation. Examples are provided in Figure 5.

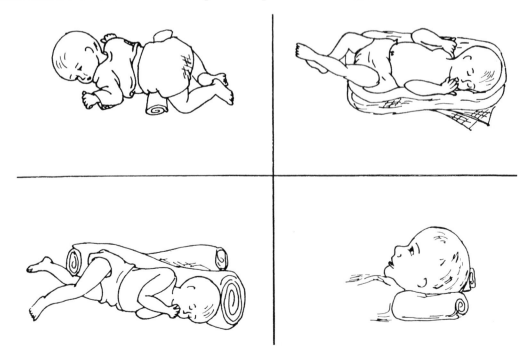

Figure 5. Positioning alternatives for the premature infant   31

Sensorimotor Activities

With a baby in the NICU, the therapist uses tactile, vestibular, proprioceptive, visual and auditory stimuli to assist the infant in achieving maximal interaction with caregivers and to facilitate the experience of normal postural and movement patterns.

Swaddling is a form of tactile stimulation that is valuable in promoting flexion and midline orientation. Use of swaddling helps to decrease irritability. It is especially useful during medical interventions and feeding [Figure 6].

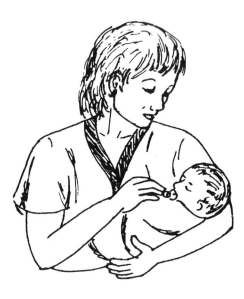

Figure 6. Swaddling

Movement providing vestibular input can be extremely helpful with the premature infant. Slow, repetitive movement in a vertical direction can soothe and calm an irritable infant. Quicker movements or more abrupt movements in the horizontal plane can be arousing. Swaddling during movement provides additional tactile input to assist in calming the baby. It is important to maintain a flexed position during these maneuvers. Older babies may tolerate more vigorous movement experiences such as rhythmical bouncing when held at your shoulder or rocking in a horizontal direction. During movement experiences, careful monitoring of physiologic stress signs is very important. The proper use of these sensorimotor activities enhances the infant's opportunities for early movement experiences.

In addition to the positioning and sensorimotor techniques described above, there are three important sensorimotor activities that can be incorporated into routine caregiving. First, caregivers can facilitate head lifting by sitting the infant up when burping during feeding [Figure 7-a]. Second, caregivers can decrease hypertonicity in the legs during a diaper change by gently rocking the baby's pelvis

[Figure 7-b]. Third, shoulder retraction can be inhibited by providing weight bearing on the shoulders during diapering [Figure 7-c].

Figure 7.

Routine caregiving using sensorimotor activities

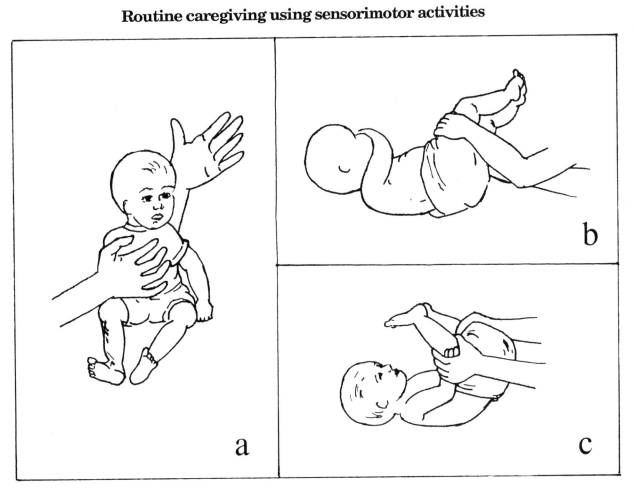

Figure 7-a. Facilitating head lifting when burping

Figure 7-b . Decreasing lower extremity hypertonicity during diaper change

Figure 7-c. Inhibiting shoulder retraction during diaper change

A number of ***feeding strategies*** may be helpful in resolving the feeding difficulties common among the high risk infants. The weak and uncoordinated suck-swallow mechanism, the long term use of the endotracheal tube, and the high expenditure of energy during oral feeding often contribute to feeding problems. One of the best documented techniques for improving nutritional status is the use of non-nutritive sucking. Providing an infant with a pacifier during gavage feeding has been shown to improve weight gain by improving digestion (Measel & Anderson, 1979) and behavioral state control (Neely, 1979). Also, the opportunity to suck may strengthen oral musculature (Harris, 1986). Other techniques for improving feeding include tactile stimulation to the oral musculature during feeding, along with jaw stabilization and maintenance of a midline head position with a chin tuck and semiflexed positioning [Figure 8].

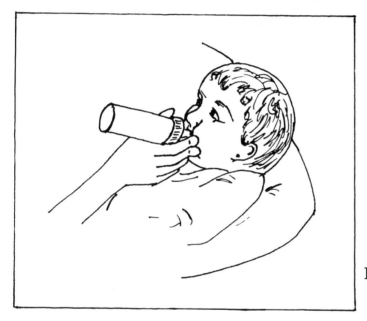

Figure 8. Positioning for feeding

Parents and Therapeutic Intervention

For intervention to be effective, the therapist must work with parents and the nursing staff. In teaching parents handling techniques, the therapist should be as clear and concise as possible. Terminology and jargon should be kept to a minimum and explained fully. Written guidelines and pictures individualized to each baby can be tremendously important and can improve parents' overall skills and understanding of their child's needs. Meeting with parents on a regular basis to teach only one or two developmental tasks at a time can be an effective method in promoting parental understanding and enthusiasm in carrying out recommendations.

Because parents' visiting hours may not routinely overlap with the therapist's visits to the NICU, a variety of ***communication strategies*** are needed. Posting developmental cards on the isolette or maintaining a communication book are two effective methods for keeping parents abreast of the developmental program. It is important that new cards be posted regularly even if only small changes are made in the program so that parents do not become discouraged performing the same activities over a long period. Therapists should be sensitive to the individual family's level of emotional and physical stress and adjust accordingly their expectations regarding involvement with the therapeutic program.

Staff Education

Pediatric therapists expecting follow up and support of developmental activities must be involved in ongoing communication with nursery staff. Formal in-service programs on the developmental needs of preterm infants, positioning techniques, and oral-motor facilitation strategies should be provided to the nursing and medical staff. Also, therapists must be flexible in scheduling inservice programs and demonstrations. Staffing patterns of special care nurseries do not easily lend themselves to traditional inservice programming. To gain acceptance as an integral part of the NICU team, therapists must be available to fit the needs of the nursery staff.

Individualized follow up instruction for specific strategies for particular babies is also needed. Therapists will need to communicate to the primary caregivers of individual babies concerning recommendations and to clarify concerns and questions. However, therapists should appreciate that nurses may have many competing demands and may have difficulty following through with developmental activities. The activities and/or strategies should be designed to be incorporated into the daily nursing care plan and should be taught from that framework.

Summary

Physical and occupational therapists continue to increase their involvement in the NICU. The information provided here describes the basic components of an effective therapeutic treatment program for infants in the NICU. Pediatric therapists have much to offer this very special population of infants. However, therapists must be prepared to design comprehensive treatment programs based on sound scientific principles which can lead to professional accountability. Programs must be presented in a format that is understandable to the infant's primary nursing team as well as to parents. When comprehensive treatment programs are developed in this context, the infants, families, and NICU staff have much to gain.

3 MOVING FAMILIES TOWARD INDEPENDENT CAREGIVING: THE DISCHARGE PHASE

Successful transition to home care can only be achieved when discharge is viewed as part of an ongoing process that begins at the time of the infant's birth. The ultimate objective of this process is the fostering of parental competence and confidence in their ability to manage the medical and developmental needs of their chronically ill or medically fragile infant. Emphasis in the period immediately prior to discharge must be placed on helping families assume an independent role in managing their infant's needs.

PREPARATION FOR DISCHARGE

Once the child's medical status has stabilized, the transition to home management can be considered. An initial step in preparation for discharge is assessment of the major areas that will impact on the family's ability to care for the infant at home. These include:

- the infant's medical and developmental status,
- family strengths and needs,
- the physical home environment, and
- community resources.

Specific assessment procedures and considerations regarding each of these areas are described below.

Assessment of the Infant's Status

The level of medical caregiving that the infant will require is a primary factor in determining the feasibility of home management. This is an important first step in the assessment process. The neonatologist and nursing staff evaluate, as a minimum:

- the level of respiratory support that the infant needs,
- the feeding method and rate of weight gain,
- the infant's autonomic regulation including respiration, heart rate and body temperature, and
- medication needs.

By gathering this information, the medical and nursing staff can determine what home equipment needs exist and what specific skill training the parents will need. The amount of time needed to secure necessary equipment and prepare parents also plays a role in determining the discharge date.

The nursery staff usually develops a list of home equipment and supplies that will be needed. At Georgetown University Hospital, the NICU social worker is responsible for assisting the family in making arrangements with equipment suppliers and home health care personnel. The developmental team nurse can provide a supportive role in assisting the social worker and family in arranging the complex health services often needed for home management of the chronically ill infant.

The infant's developmental status may also play a role in determining the services needed post discharge. Assessment of the infant's sensory status including vision and hearing should be done prior to discharge to help determine necessary follow up medical specialty services as well as rehabilitative needs. Assessment tools for determining developmental status are discussed in previous sections.

Assessment of the Family

Assessment of the family begins with evaluation of the family's motivation and willingness to care for their medically fragile infant at home. This must be based on a realistic idea of what the home care will entail. The next goal is assessment of the parents' ability to carry out caregiving needs. This includes basic caregiving functions including handling, bathing, dressing, and feeding. For many medically fragile infants it also includes:

- administration of medications.
- use of various monitoring equipment, and
- cardiopulmonary resuscitation,

For some chronically ill infants it may also require:

- use of oxygen equipment and suctioning procedures,
- gavage or gastrostomy feeding, and
- tracheostomy care.

The complexity of caregiving demands, therefore, depends on the infant's medical condition.

Basic caregiving skills are usually assessed informally. For children with complex medical needs, specific checklists have been developed to assess caregiver competence. *A Skills Checklist for Individuals Caring for the Child Who is Tracheostomized and/or Ventilator Assisted* from the Georgetown University Rainbow Series manual on *The Family As Care Manager: Home Care Coordination for Medically Fragile Children* written by Kaufman and Lichtenstein is included in Figure 9. *The Needs Assessment for Home Care*, by the same authors, is a parent-reported needs assessment from the same Rainbow series manual and is included in Figure 10. The parent's own report of needs is a basic element in service delivery that is truly family-centered. This needs assessment checklist might be given to families to complete early in the discharge planning process. An updating of needs can occur just prior to discharge and again shortly after discharge.

Other factors beyond parental caretaking competency may affect the family's ability to manage the child at home. Family stresses such as need for sibling care, financial need, and respite care needs may make it difficult for a competent and well intentioned parent to successfully manage a chronically ill child at home. These potential sources of stress need to be explored. While the neonatologist has basic responsibility for determining medical needs, the developmental team, working with hospital social workers, can support families in recognizing these non-medical needs and collaboratively seeking solutions for them.

Figure 9

**Skills Checklist for Individuals Caring for the Child
Who Is Tracheostomized and/or Ventilator Assisted**
Coordinating Center for Home and Community Care, Inc.

	Date Describe	Date Demo
Annual Pediatric CPR Certification	_____	
Annual Malpractice Insurance	_____	
Client Confidentiality Issues Discussed	_____	

Assessments:
Breath Sounds - Auscultation:
- Before Suction
- After Suction
- Need for Aerosol

Assessment Related to Physician
Notification Orders
- Specify:

Signs and Symptoms:
- Respiratory Distress
- Hypoxia
- Side Effects of Medications
- Fluid Retention

Procedures:
Chest Physical Therapy
Suctioning:
- Positioning for
- Nasopharyngeally
- Tracheal

Trach Care:
- Clean Trach Site
- Change Trach Site
- Change Trach Tube
- Cleaning of Inner Cannula
- Place on Trach Collar

Bagging:
- Via Trach
- Via Mouth

(Reprinted by permission from Kaufman, J. and Lichtenstein, K.A., The Family as Care Manager: Home Care Coordination for Medically Fragile Children. Washington, D.C.: Georgetown University Child Development Center)

Skills Checklist for Individuals Caring for Child (continued - page 2)

Emergency Protocol/Procedure   _____
* Knowledge of   _____
* "Mock" Demonstration   _____

Monitoring and Equipment:
Vital Signs   _____
Skin Care   _____
Oral Hygiene   _____
Use of Apnea/Bradycardia Monitor   _____

Check Monitor Settings/Check Monitor Alarm
     Systems   _____
Use of Lead Wires/Placement of Child   _____
Use of Belt/Placement of Child   _____

Placement on Oxygen Delivery Device/Trach
     Collar   _____
Placement of Ventilator   _____
Calibrate Oxygen Analyzer   _____
Check Oxygen Level/Liter Flow   _____
Check Oxygen Tank Level   _____
Check/Calibrate Ventilator Settings   _____
* IMV   _____
* PEEP   _____
* Pressure Units   _____
* Tidal Volume   _____
Systematic Troubleshooting of Ventilator   _____
Use of Respirometer   _____
Humidity System:
* Check Water Level   _____
* Check Temperature   _____
* Filling Procedure   _____
* Draining Water from Tubing   _____
* Cleaning of Humidity Bottles/Cascade   _____
Check Compressor Operation   _____
Clean Compressor Unit Screen   _____
Assess Suction Machine Pressure   _____
Clean Suction Machine   _____
Clean Suction Catheters   _____
Clean Corrugated Tubing   _____
Clean Manual Resuscitation Device
     (Reservoir Bag & Associated Equip)   _____
Clean Trach Collar   _____
Clean Trach Tubes   _____
* Disposable   _____
* Metal   _____

Skills Checklist for Individuals Caring for Child (continued - page 3)

Medication Administration:
Action and Side Effects   _____
Normal Dosage   _____
Administration Techniques (as appropriate)   _____
Documentation   _____
Installation of Normal Saline   _____
Administration of Aerosol Treatments   _____

Documentation:
Activity Level   _____
Observations/Respiratory Distress   _____
Nursing Procedures   _____
Safety Protocol   _____
Equipment Checks and Cleaning   _____
Transport Protocol
    • Emergency   _____
    • Non-Emergency   _____

Additional Individualized Assessment/Skills

_____   _____
_____   _____
_____   _____
_____   _____
_____   _____
_____   _____

Please Indicate N/A when Nonapplicable

I (Supervisor/Designee), _____have inserviced the individual designated as Orientee regarding assessments and skills listed above.

Initial and Date indicates procedure has been described and/or demonstrated in a competent manner.

I (Orientee), _____understand all assessments and skills listed above and am able to perform same in a competent and confident manner.

Child's Name _____
Physician _____
      Phone _____

Figure 10

Needs Assessment for Home Care
Coordinating Center for Home and Community Care, Inc.

1. Will you need safety equipment in your home?
   Smoke detector   _____
   Fire extinguisher   _____
   Other_____

2. Will you need adaptions in your home?   _____
   Ramping   _____
   Bathroom changes   _____
   Other_____

3. Will you need adaptive equipment?
   Wheelchair   _____
   Travel safety seat   _____
   Stroller   _____
   Other_____

4. Will your utilities need updating?
   Air conditioner   _____
   Humidifier   _____
   Heat   _____
   Electricity (circuitry)   _____
   Electricity (3 prong outlets)   _____
   Generator   _____
   Other_____

5. Do you need a telephone?   _____

6. Do you know who to call in case of emergency?   _____

7. Do you need to plan for your other children in case you have
   to leave quickly?   _____

8. Do you need to plan for your disabled child in case you have
   to leave quickly?   _____

9. Do you need to plan for child care in case of your own illness? _____

10. Do you need an alternative caregiver?   _____

11. Will you need assistance with transportation?   _____

12. Will you need assistance in locating child care for your other
    children?   _____

13. Will you need assistance with household chores?   _____

(Reprinted by permission from Kaufman, J. and Lichtenstein, K.A., The Family as Care Manager: Home Care Coordination for Medically Fragile Children. Washington, D.C.: Georgetown University Child Development Center)

Needs Assessment for Home Care (continued - page 2)

14. Do you need to make any changes in your home environment that have not been mentioned? _____

15. Do you need to plan for respite care? _____

16. Do you need a local pediatrician for well baby care? _____
    Name:_____

17. Do you need a specialty physician or clinic to follow your child? _____

18. Do you need help locating a pharmacist? _____

19. Do you need a source for formula? _____

20. Do you need assistance in locating/ordering everyday baby supplies? _____

21. Do you need additional training in your child's care? _____

22. Do you need more information about your child's condition? _____

23. Do you need therapies for your child in your home?
    OT _____
    PT _____
    Speech _____

24. Do alternate caregivers still need training? _____

25. Do you need specific guidelines for your child's readmission to the hospital? _____

26. Do you need specific guidelines for when to call the physician?_____

27. Do you need to be trained in CPR (cardiopulmonary resuscitation)? _____

28. Do alternate caregivers need to be trained in CPR? _____

29. Do you need instruction in the care and use of equipment in your home? _____

30. Do you need guidelines for dealing with specific problems you have with your equipment vendor? _____

31. Do you need updated educational evaluations? _____

32. Will your child need a referral for Child Find/Infant Stimulation? _____

33. Will you need shifts of nursing in your home? _____

34. Do you need assistance in selecting an agency? _____

35. If you have nurses in your home, do you need guidelines for dealing with specific problems? _____

36. Do you need assistance with scheduling nursing? _____

Needs Assessment for Home Care (continued - page 3)

37. Do you want a referral to a parent support group or would you like to talk to another parent?   _____

38. Do you need a referral for counseling?
    Individual   _____
    Marital   _____
    Family   _____
    Child   _____

39. Do you need more information about your insurance coverage?_____

40. Do you need more information about/or applications for public programs?

WIC	_____	Section 8	_____
SSI	_____	Sub. Housing	_____
M A	_____	Energy Assist. Prog.	_____
Waiver	_____	Crippled Children's	_____
AFDC	_____		

41. Will you need articles for your child prior to homecoming?

Toys	_____	Age	_____
Clothing	_____	Size	_____
Car Seat	_____		
Crib	_____		
Equipment	_____		

42. Will you need assistance with your finances and budget?   _____

43. Are there needs you are concerned about which have not been mentioned?   _____

Home Environment Assessment

A home visit prior to discharge should be arranged to determine whether there is a need to adapt the physical environment in order to manage the child at home. There must be adequate *space for equipment* the child might need. Safety issues such as fire exits can also be noted at this time. For children who are technology dependent, the existence of *adequate electrical supply* to handle the medical equipment should be determined. Access to a *telephone* and *alarms indicating smoke or power failure* emergencies may also be necessary.

A Physical Facility Checklist for the Home from the Georgetown University Rainbow Series manual on *Getting Children Home: Hospital to Community,* written by Bilotti, is included in Figure 11.

Recommendations for adapting the environment to facilitate home management of the child can be made based on the information gathered during the visit.

Figure 11

Physical Facility Checklist for the Home
Children's Home Health Network of Illinois

Hospital _____ City_____ Date_____

Patient's Name_____ Hospital I.D.#_____

Prepared By_____ Title_____ Telephone_____

Physical Facility Standards for the Home	**Satisfactory**	**Unsatisfactory**

I. Accessibility

A. Physical facility must accommodate the child's specific disability (to include) equipment necessary for facilitating mobility and/or transport) to provide access with single caretaker assistance.

B. Where applicable, physical facility must not restrict delivery of large or heavy medical equipment.

II. Space Requirements

A. Child's room must have minimum square footage area of 9 ft.x 9 ft.
   Note: Any living areas in the house may be designated as the "child's room" (e.g., bedroom, dining room, recreation room).

B. **Storage**

   1. **Immediate access**, e.g., night stand-- used to store equipment/supplies with utilization frequency of 8 hrs. or less, e.g., suction catheters, suction machine, gloves, dropper bottle.

   2. **Proximal access**, e.g., closet--used to store equipment/supplies with utilization frequency of 24 hrs. or less, e.g., infant scale, water bottles, specimen cups, and immediate access items in larger quantities. Can include small volumes of oxygen replacement. The proximal access storage area must be in close proximity to the child's room.

(Reprinted by permission from Bilotti, G. Getting Children Home: Hospital to Community. Washington, D.C.: Georgetown University Child Development Center)

Physical Facility Checklist for the Home (continued - page 2)

Satisfactory   Unsatisfactory

3. **Bulk storage,** e.g., basement or garage--
   must be large enough to accommodate 1
   month's equipment/supplies and at
   least 1 week's oxygen supply.
   Storage areas must be free from excessive dampness. The temperature must
   not permit water to freeze. Storage
   areas must not contain toxic chemicals,
   e.g., cleaning solutions, fertilizer.

III. Electricity Requirements

A. A qualified electrician is required to
    evaluate the physical facility for ability
    to accommodate the child's electrical
    supply needs.

B. The physical facility must be supplied by
    a minimum of 100 amp. electrical service.

C. A minimum of two separate 15 amp. branch
    circuits must supply the child's room.

D. If the main distribution panel utilizes fuses,
    four spare fuses of appropriate capacity are
    required to be stored near the fuse box.

E. A minimum of four duplex electrical
    outlets on each of the two 15 amp. branch
    circuits is required for a total of eight
    duplex outlets in the child's room.
    Note: This is in addition to the usual and
          customary installation.Therefore,
          this requirement is not to be inter-
          preted as the total number of outlets
          required by the child's room.

IV. Special Equipment

A. A telephone should be at the child's
    bedside.

B. A mechanical whistle should be at the
    child's bedside.

C. A battery-powered fluorescent flood
    light should be at the child's bedside.

Physical Facility Checklist for the Home (continued - page 3)

Satisfactory   Unsatisfactory

D.   Power failure alarm/light should be plugged into the same house electrical circuit as the ventilator.

E.   One smoke alarm and one five pound CO_2 fire extinguisher should be located on each level of the home (including the basement).

V.   Ventilation

A.   Ventilation must be adequate to permit safe recharging of wet cell marine type batteries.

B.   Oxygen storage areas must have adequate ventilation.

VI.   General

The house must meet local safety, sanitation, and building requirements.

VII.   Other Considerations

VIII.   Summary of equipment/home modifications necessary for safe discharge home:

Assessment of Community Resource Needs

Families of chronically ill infants typically need a number of support services from community agencies once their child is discharged home. Those with infants with complex needs, especially technology dependent infants, will require a variety of community resources. Among those resources often needed are:

- a primary physician experienced in medical needs of chronically ill infants,
- Visiting Nurse Association home visitor,
- home nursing care agency,
- medical equipment company,
- rescue squad availability,
- a nearby medical care facility,
- electrical company power-failure emergency alert,
- developmental intervention team,
- trained child care provider, and
- respite care

Availability of these services should be explored during discharge planning in order that appropriate notification can be given to relevant agencies.

Throughout this predischarge assessment phase, developmental staff can work closely with families in assisting them to articulate and prioritize their own needs. Interdisciplinary input from the various team members is useful in developing solutions to problems that arise. At times, needs apparent to the professionals may not be considered relevant by the families. If collaborative goal setting between parents and professionals is to exist, professionals may need to accept a family's unwillingness to address a particular need at a certain point in time. *Only when professionals respect the individual family's priorities does an equal partnership exist between families and professionals.*

DISCHARGE CONFERENCE

Once post discharge needs have been assessed, a discharge planning conference may be scheduled by the attending physician. Participants at the conference will usually include:

- parents,
- neonatologists,
- primary nurse,
- primary physician,
- developmental team case manager,
- developmental team nurse or discharge nurse.

The purpose of this conference is to determine tasks to be accomplished prior to discharge and needs to be addressed after discharge.

It is helpful if the conference begins with a *general overview* of the infant's hospital course. Some prediction may be offered as to the child's expected medical course over the ensuing weeks. *Results of the various assessments* conducted during the preparation phase can then be shared with the family. This might include a summary of the child's developmental status and a self report of family concerns as described to the social worker and on the self report questionnaire. The family may then further elaborate on their perception of needs. Parents are encouraged to ask questions to insure that all areas of their infant's home care are understood. Typical questions raised by families include health risk issues such as exposure to visitors or individuals outside the home and concerns related to sleeping and feeding.

Necessary *post discharge medical care and developmental follow up* can be discussed and responsibility assigned for scheduling of appointments. Areas of caregiving in which parents may need more training can also be discussed and arrangements made for providing such training. A discharge planning conference conducted in this way results in a list of discharge needs with an individual identified to assist in meeting each need and a timeline proposed for completion of each task. See Figure 12 for an example of a discharge plan.

ACTIVITIES PRIOR TO DISCHARGE

Activities necessary for meeting the needs of the discharge plan are pursued during the period prior to discharge. Arrangements for purchasing or leasing of necessary home equipment will need to be made. Community support services should be made aware of the discharge timeframe and date for implementation of services. In addition, parent training in areas such as feeding and respiratory management can now move toward completion. The medical staff has ultimate responsibility for approving the level of competence achieved by the parent for adequately meeting the infant's health needs. Developmental staff can assist in helping the parents build confidence in their skills by being available during caregiving practice sessions and giving feedback to the parents.

It may be helpful to have the parents stay for an overnight period toward the end of this phase to assume full caregiving responsibility. This provides them an opportunity to demonstrate their capability for managing needs with nursing support nearby. Some families may choose to do this for more than one night.

In some instances, preparing a parent for home caregiving may require a more extended training period. Young single mothers who have had limited family support and little caregiving experience with full-term healthy infants may require more assistance prior to discharge in order to prepare them to raise a medically fragile child. Training these mothers to understand medical regimes such as apnea monitoring, suctioning, and administration of various medications may be a gradual process. The mothers may be helped by weekend visits to practice supervised caregiving for their infants. Developmental staff can participate in these training sessions and make home visits in order to garner further extended family support to assist these mothers in their caregiving responsibilities at home.

Figure 12

DISCHARGE PLAN
Self Care Needs

Patient: D.H.

Anticipated Discharge: **7/10/88**

Primary Nursing Team: **LL, SS, LH**

Discharge Needs	Staff	Anticipated Date	Actual Date of Completion
Sleep study scheduled	SS	7/1/88	7/1/88
CPR/monitor training completed	LL	7/5/88	7/5/88 7/6/88
Parents verbalize knowledge of apnea/bradycardia, color changes, false alarms, safety measures and medications	LL/LH	7/5/88 7/6/88	7/5/88 7/6/88
Parents able to administer medication safely	SS/LH	7/7/88	7/7/88
Parents able to bathe, feed handle, wrap, provide circumcision care and diaper infant	LL/SS	7/1/88	7/3/88
Parents able to verbalize principles of infant care	LL/SS/LH	7/5/88	7/5/88
Parents have car seat available	LL	7/8/88	7/7/88
Parents aware of post discharge appointments:	LL		
ophthalmologist		7/15/88	
primary pediatrician		7/11/88	
DEC follow up		8/13/88	
Apnea clinic		7/18/88	

Infant feeding is an especially critical area for monitoring by both NICU nurses and developmental staff. The feeding interaction provides an important opportunity for parents to become sensitive to their infant's response patterns. A parent's sense of competence in parenting their infant may be closely linked with a successful feeding experience. The parent may need support in achieving a mutually satisfying feeding interaction especially with an infant who is irritable or who tires easily. The parent's availability during a 24 hour period will allow close observation by intervention staff of the feeding interaction.

Parents can be encouraged to get plenty of rest the evening before discharge. They may be encouraged to do something relaxing for themselves such as go out to dinner the night before discharge. This special treat will help them support each other as they begin what is often the very difficult period of home care.

The procedure in Georgetown University Hospital's NICU on the day of discharge begins with the parent or parents being met in the nursery by the primary nurse and neonatologist. The discharge plan is reviewed and any final questions addressed. A follow up phone call is made to the family by the primary nurse that evening to provide support and encouragement and answer any further questions. Just prior to discharge the developmental team nurse schedules an initial post discharge home visit to occur during the infant's first week at home.

HOME CARE MANAGEMENT

During the first post-discharge week, it is helpful if the team nurse can conduct daily follow up calls and at least one home visit. During this visit, caregiving needs can be reviewed and any areas of concern regarding caregiving can be addressed. In addition, a physical exam of the infant can be conducted and baseline growth parameters collected. Further appointments can also be discussed, and developmental suggestions such as calming techniques for the infant reviewed. Parents should be encouraged to discuss any area causing concerns at this time, including those not directly related to infant caregiving.

Consideration should also be given to conducting a second home visit by the second post-discharge week. After the child has been home a few weeks, the case manager can conduct a family-focused interview to determine family strengths and needs. Further discussion of the family-focused interview appears in the next section: **Maintaining a Family- Centered Approach**.

SUMMARY

Successful transition to home care is dependent on good discharge planning and parent preparation. Careful assessment of the infant's health needs and family and community resources available for meeting those needs is essential. Preparation of parents in the skills needed for home management of the infant will help assure continued infant development and allow parents to feel competent in themselves caring for their infant. The family's own perception of their needs and priorities in the transition to home care is a major consideration if home care is to be successful. Coordination of needed community services will result in reduced family stress and more optimum health status for the infant.

4 MAINTAINING A FAMILY-CENTERED APPROACH

There has been an evolution in the nature and form of early intervention services. This evolution moved from a focus on the infants themselves as the primary target for intervention to an emphasis on the mother-infant dyad as the target. There is now a third stage which recognizes the importance of the family as collaborators in the intervention process.

This gradual shift in emphasis from infant to mother-infant to family-infant has resulted, in part, from the recognition of the importance of the family's role in the development of the infant, including infants with specific biological risks. The developmental process is dynamic with characteristics of the infant, family, and greater environment reciprocally affecting one another over time. If we are to improve outcome for the infant, we must impact on each of the areas that contribute to developmental progress in the infant.

Earlier approaches to intervention conceived of the relationship of professionals with the family as "doing to" the family. We have entered a new philosophical approach in which families and professionals *serve as partners* in formulation of goals and implementation of intervention strategies.

AREAS OF FAMILY NEED

For improved outcome, needs of both the family and the infant must be addressed. The framework used by the authors follows that of Bailey and Simeonsson (1984), who identify three family needs which the authors see across families of at risk or handicapped children. These three needs are:

1. A *means for coping with the stress* imposed by having an at risk or chronically ill infant.
2. A *method for establishing control* within an environment where the families perceive they have no control.
3. *Building quality interactions* with their at risk or chronically ill infant.

As part of the shift in parent-professional relationships, new emphasis is placed on family-centered intervention. In recognition of the importance of the family's role in successful intervention, the family's own view of their needs becomes an important part of intervention planning. Families and professionals work collaboratively to identify needs and prioritize objectives.

Families' Coping with Stress

The first few months following the birth of an at risk or handicapped infant are likely to be highly stressful for families due to the fragile medical status of the infant and the often uncertain prognosis. When the infant is acutely ill and hospitalized for a prolonged period of time, parents' resources can be taxed and parent-infant attachment impeded.

Families of at risk and handicapped infants, and members within these families, cope with the stresses of this period in differing ways. Interventionists must be aware of different coping mechanisms, including needs for denial or displacement, and develop an appreciation for each family's unique style of coping. Additionally, members within a family may cope in different ways. One member may be very direct with feelings, another, withholding. In a number of families, we have noted that men and women often employ different approaches. While the stereotypic pattern is for women to be more comfortable and direct with emotional expression, this pattern is not characteristic in all families. Another typical pattern is for one member of the family to be the optimist and the other to adopt a pessimistic stance. Service providers must understand and accept these differences and help family members to do the same for each other. The interventionist must also recognize the unique set of social and cultural values that will affect a particular family's functioning.

Appreciation for Family Systems

A useful framework for describing and interpreting family needs is found in family systems theory. Systems theory emphasizes interpreting family needs, values, and priorities within the context of the family's own system (e.g., resources, functions, interactional patterns) and societal system (e.g., neighborhoods, cultural groups, prevailing social attitudes). Recognizing the impact of systems factors may lead to a greater understanding of the family's perspective; it may also help interventionists anticipate the possible impact of treatment recommendations on the infant as well as the larger system. As an example, in some families and cultural groups, problems are to be kept private and solutions found within the family. Having to turn to professionals and expose private matters to someone outside the family may be difficult for some families to accept.

Appreciation for Competing Needs

Professionals often formulate their own ideas as to the services the family needs, the priorities a family should adopt, or the behaviors which parents should demonstrate during the NICU course. For instance, staff may believe that parents of infants in the NICU should visit often, should not show anger or be difficult, and should have an understanding of complex medical concepts. Intervention staff must try to be aware of, understand, and empathize with each individual family's response to the NICU experience.

We have found, for example, that some families may not be able to visit often because of transportation problems or difficulty obtaining child care for other siblings. Anger may be exhibited by parents as a common part of the grieving process and must be acknowledged as a necessary reaction. Each parent's educational background and stage in the grief process may effect how rapidly medical information is absorbed.

Support must be offered that addresses the need of an individual family or member of a family; support is not offered according to a preset plan. For instance, a family may need a variety of community support services before they are ready to deal emotionally with their infant. The interventionist might assist parents in obtaining transportation, housing, food stamps, or SSI which the parent might see as priorities above the needs for enhancing parent-infant interaction.

Families' Need for a Sense of Control

The experience of having a critically ill infant often results in parents feeling powerless over their fate. Experiences that allow a family to regain a sense of equilibrium and personal control are helpful.

During the NICU phase, the family may be taught to recognize the infant's response patterns. They then may be helped to explore ways in which their handling of the infant promotes greater autonomic stability in the infant. Parents may feel a greater sense of control when their own observations are acknowledged and have an impact. Ultimately, parents feel the greatest sense of control when they can serve as care provider and protector for their infant. This is a gradual process in which professionals can help families to develop knowledge and skills that will allow their functioning in this role. Families also will vary in the degree of control they may want to maintain, at different points in time, in decision making in regards to their infant's needs.

Families' Need for Quality Interactions With Their Infants

Successful interactions with their infants also are a means for families to experience a sense of control. The development of mutually satisfying interactions between chronically ill infants and their families is a gradual process. When the infants are acutely ill, they may be intolerant of or unavailable for interaction. This is difficult for parents who want to hold and care for their own infant.

Teaching parents to recognize times when the infant may be alert and ready for interaction may be helpful in their feelings that they are getting to "know" their infant. Chronically ill infants may often demonstrate irritability. Here, again, if parents know ways in which to soothe the infant, they may feel more successful in parenting their infant. *Understanding My Signals: Help for Parents of Premature Infants* (Hussey, 1988) is a booklet designed to provide parents with this type of information. The developmental intervention team uses both written materials and direct observation to promote enhanced parent-child interaction throughout the hospital course and after discharge.

Families' Need for Peer Support

While support from hospital staff is of benefit to most families, parents often find a special kind of support from other parents who have experienced similar problems.

Georgetown University Hospital has a "Parents of Premies" group made up of parents of current or former NICU babies, offering regular meetings for families. Families of new arrivals in the NICU are made aware of the group meetings and are usually contacted by one of the group members. Membership in the parent group fluctuates. Families tend to be most active in their participation while the infant is hospitalized and during the first year after discharge. Some families have remained active for many years in the organization and serve to provide direction and continuity in the group.

Other hospitals use parent-to-parent support networks in which trained parents of former NICU babies are available for support to newer parents. These groups provide support to newer families in additional ways besides information and emotional support. Sometimes parents may work out carpools to assist families with transportation problems to visit the infant. Other families may open their homes for overnight stays to parents of current NICU babies, especially if the parents reside far from the hospital.

There are other specific situations in the lives of families of chronically ill infants in which peer support is particularly helpful. For example, parents of a terminally ill baby may benefit from talking with parents of another baby who has died. Parents of a baby requiring a particular medical procedure may find help by being in touch with parents of a baby who has successfully undergone the same procedure. The hospital staff can be supportive of these parent-to-parent efforts by providing a meeting place and serving as resources for needed information.

FAMILY-FOCUSED INTERVENTION IN THE NICU

In order to identify family needs, an *assessment of family functioning* early in the care process is essential. Information must be gathered from the family, the social worker, and nurses on psychosocial risk factors that may adversely impact on the family system, parental attitudes/perceptions about the infant, and the family support systems.

As the chronically ill infant's health status stabilizes, developmental staff can assess and foster an increasingly active parental role in caregiving. Parents participate in feeding and other caregiving tasks on a regular basis, and they are encouraged to stay overnight at the hospital in preparation for assuming full responsibility for their infant (e.g., diapering, bathing, dressing, feeding, suctioning). During these interactions the NICU and developmental staff can assist the parents in refining their skills to carry out these tasks. Parent input of their own feelings of competence should also be encouraged. This evolving process of setting gradual expectations for increased parental caregiving facilitates more positive parental perceptions of the infant and greater competence in managing the infant's needs.

FAMILY-FOCUSED INTERVENTION AT DISCHARGE

It is important to begin assessing the family's individual post-discharge needs prior to discharge. The theoretical framework underlying the family-focused assessment used by the authors originates from the F.A.M.I.L.I.E.S. project of the Frank Porter Graham Center for Child Development at the University of North Carolina, Chapel Hill (Bailey et al, 1986). Within the model, the perceptions of both family and interventionist are given similar value in the development of an intervention plan. Therefore, assessments incorporate self-rating and self-report activities by parents as well as observations by staff members. A number of assessment tools used in the F.A.M.I.L.I.E.S. project have been incorporated into procedures used for chronically ill infants. These include:

- a Survey of Family Needs,
- a Parent Knowledge Survey, and
- the Nowicki-Strickland Measure of Locus of Control.

Four dimensions of family functioning need to be assessed. These include:
- *child variables* - child responsiveness, temperament, caregiving demands;
- *parent variables* - personal beliefs, stress, sources of support;
- *parent-child interaction* - reading and responding to infant cues, attachment relationship; and
- *family needs* - information, informal and formal support, community services, finances.

Data regarding family needs can be obtained during the period when discharge preparation has begun. This allows development of a management plan to meet infant and family needs during the preparation for discharge and after discharge. It is useful for interdisciplinary team members to conduct weekly staffings to discuss assessment data obtained by each family's case manager. The case manager can explore with the family all areas that may impact on the family's ability to cope and provide care for the infant. In this way, assessment information remains family-focused and goes beyond addressing only the needs of the infant as perceived by the staff.

Family-Focused Interview

A full family-focused interview can be conducted approximately two to three weeks after the infant has been discharged home from the hospital. This interview model also originates from the F.A.M.I.L.I.E.S. project (Winton and Bailey, 1988). It is helpful to conduct this interview after the discharge primarily because the family will be able to better determine their needs once they have had the opportunity to manage their infant at home. This provides a time to resolve any conflicts that have arisen and hopefully prevent further ones. The family can be asked to assemble those family members who will be involved in management of the infant. The meeting is then scheduled in the home at a convenient time.

The family-focused interviewer should review the assessment material and develop a preliminary outline of some of the specific areas of concern to be discussed prior to the meeting. During the interview itself, however, it is important for interventionists to listen to families identify additional areas of concern. The interviewer must respond empathically to family concerns, follow feelings expressed by family members, probe the details in a sensitive fashion, utilize both open and closed-ended questions, focus in depth on issues of particular concern and help families recognize their strengths.

The interview follows a general sequence that includes:

- an introduction explaining the purpose and format of the interview
- discussion of the family's strengths and needs
- summary and prioritization of intervention goals
- discussion of tasks to be completed and who will be responsible
- time for response to remaining questions and closure.

It is important for the interviewer to *facilitate* but not direct the discussion. The family should be encouraged to assume the lead role. This will require the interviewer to have skills in presenting questions in an open ended way, allowing the family to guide the direction of elaboration to questions. The interviewer must use sensitivity in eliciting discussion about family relationships with reassurance to the family about confidentiality of issues that would be discussed.

While the family may be direct in suggesting particular needs that would be met through the intervention plan, the interviewer may need to listen during the discussion for what may be problems for the family that they have not yet identified or verbalized. The interviewer might then try to restate those concerns as a formal need and have the family discuss whether that need exists and where they might place it on a list of priorities.

Potential needs can be identified through the discussion as well as through previously obtained family and infant assessment measures. A variety of information sources is thus drawn upon to provide a comprehensive picture of family and infant functioning.

During the interview, the interventionist and the family engage in a process of identifying and negotiating goals. Conflicts in goal perception must be recognized and attempts made to resolve them. When a conflict exists, Bailey (1987) recommends that the interventionist and family try to reach agreement on a practical issue. This negotiation often involves the consideration of multiple alternatives in an attempt to seek the best mutually acceptable solution.

Collaborative Goal-Setting

Parents not involved in setting goals for themselves may feel pressured or resistant about working toward a goal when they themselves do not regard it as a priority. In such instances, parents may give verbal agreement to a goal or activity but fail to work toward its accomplishment. A collaborative approach to goal-setting is desirable because parents are more likely to be invested in a goal or activity to which they themselves have provided input.

Professionals must also learn to accept, in this framework, that parents may not wish to work for a goal that the interventionist views as a need. With the passage of time, parents will sometimes come to see the need as the professional does. *Professionals must be flexible* to accommodate changing priorities of families as they gain more information and understanding, and as stress diminishes.

With chronically ill infants, dilemmas are sometimes presented when a parent does not perceive a health need identified by professionals as a need for their family. In these circumstances, health professionals must work to provide parents with information so that they do not endanger the health status of the infant. Further discussion of this issue appears in the section on home services.

The Individual Family Service Plan (IFSP)

Public Law 99-457 regulations provide for the development of a formal intervention plan called an **Individualized Family Service Plan (IFSP)**. The family-focused interview process described here facilitates the development of a plan to meet infant and family needs and is congruent with the intent of the IFSP as defined by P.L. 99-457. A Lead Agency has now been identified by each state to oversee development of comprehensive intervention services for at risk and handicapped children birth through two years of age. It will be important that the Lead Agency be notified of the chronically ill infant and his or her family. That agency then may be responsible for assuring a case manager for the infant's family.

COPING WITH INFANT DEATH

Because of the fragility of chronically ill infants, intervention staff occasionally find themselves in the position of providing support to families who are experiencing the death of their infant. The reality of working with this population of infants is that some will die. In some cases, the death is prolonged over several months. In other cases, the death occurs suddenly and unexpectedly. In both cases, staff can play an important role in providing support to the families of these infants.

In the case of those infants who are considered terminally ill and expected to die, staff can assist parents in working with the physicians to determine appropriate levels of care for the infant in the interim. This support will include providing explanations and answering parent's questions about guidelines for resuscitation used in the hospital. Sometimes information from the intervention team may be presented at the hospital's formal Ethics Committee meeting, the group which makes decisions about the level of extraordinary care to be provided.

Intervention staff may offer clarification about family involvement and concerns during the time the infant had been at home receiving home-based services.

As death becomes imminent for a terminally ill infant, intervention staff can provide reassurance and emotional support to the family. While medical and nursing staff are typically involved in providing intense critical care to the infant, developmental staff can spend time with parents encouraging them to hold or touch their infant and reminding them of the service they provide by remaining by their infant's side. On the other hand, if the illness lingers on and the family has other pressing needs such as children who need care at home, intervention staff can reassure the family about the appropriateness of also tending to these other concerns. Helping the family strike an appropriate balance among all the demands of their life can be reassuring for the family, and can reduce unnecessary guilt before and after the infant's death.

Intervention staff can also provide support to families whose infants die unexpectedly. This typically means establishing contact with the family by phone or in person as soon as possible after death. It is typically helpful for families to receive acknowledgement and support from individuals who knew their infant well. Often families of young chronically ill infants are somewhat isolated from extended family and family friends. This isolation may stem from prolonged hospitalization or from a natural isolation resulting from the intense caregiving needs of the chronically ill infants. Medical caregivers and developmental staff, themselves, may have filled a role as family friends, and typically form close personal relationships with the infant and family. Staff comments about the infant's unique personality and characteristics can be very meaningful to the parent whose infant has just died.

Helping the family to consider a formal memorial service can be another service provided by intervention staff. Many families may benefit from having a memorial service in their community or within the hospital. This service can help provide closure to the family on a typically stressful period in their life. This closure may be helpful for them as they begin a new phase in their life - a phase that does not carry the intense demands that are so much a part of caring for a chronically ill infant. Intervention staff may be asked to deliver a formal testimony at the memorial. Once again, expression of the personal relationship that evolves between intervention staff and individual children and their families provides a meaningful experience to families as they cope with their loss.

It should be remembered, however, that families will differ in the degree and type of support that will be most helpful to them. In one case, a mother wanted a staff member to sit with her on the PICU while her baby died in her arms. In other cases, staff provided support by sitting and talking with the family after a death, reminding them of the wonderful things about their baby - his beautiful eyes, his strong will to fight, his smile during the early days of the illness.

If intervention programs are going to provide these supports to families who experience the death of their infant, the intervention staff will have to deal with their feelings about death. It is important for staff members to be able to discuss their feelings and to provide each other with support as each person deals with the reality of death. At times, it may be necessary to have outside help to deal with the deep and sometimes contradictory feelings resulting from working with infants who die.

Work with families of chronically ill infants inevitably requires dealing with instances of infant death. Many questions are raised about the meaning and quality of life for some chronically ill infants and ethical decision-making in regards to their care. By working closely with families and listening to what families express as their needs, interventionists will be able to provide support to the family in coping with the tragedy of infant death.

SUMMARY

Effective intervention for chronically ill infants requires a family- centered focus. The family remains the best resource and advocate for the infant. The infant interventionist must work collaboratively with the family in identifying needs and setting intervention goals for the optimum benefit of both the infant and the family.

5 HOME INTERVENTION: SERVICES FOR MEDICALLY FRAGILE CHILDREN

With expanding federal mandates for provision of special education services to infants and toddlers, early intervention services are now offered in many communities. These programs are beginning to include medically fragile infants. But infants who are hospitalized for prolonged periods, or who have frequent rehospitalization, are typically unable to participate fully in these services. However, a developmental team which serves the infant both in the hospital and at home, assures that there are no gaps in service and that continuity in intervention is maintained.

Home intervention services provided by the developmental team range from direct service interventions typically provided in a community home-based intervention program to complex interagency coordination activities related to the infant's medical needs. Since the unique problems associated with serving the needs of chronically ill infants center on the latter role, this section will focus primarily on activities related to integrating medical and developmental needs.

HOME SERVICES IN THE POST-DISCHARGE PERIOD

When the medically fragile infant is discharged from the hospital, the family enters a strange new world in which their infant's very life often rests in their hands. This is an awesome responsibility for most parents. Despite good preparation prior to discharge, there is little that adequately prepares parents for the true emotional impact of leaving the NICU staff behind and being on their own.

Developmental teams can ease this transition through *information, training, and emotional support* . As described earlier, the **team nurse** plays a prominent role at discharge in assisting the family in the transition of meeting the medical caregiving needs at home. The nurse makes at least one home visit immediately after discharge and maintains daily phone contact. The case manager also visits during the first week, both to assure parents' comfort with addressing medical needs, and to help the family integrate developmental objectives into regular caregiving.

The frequency of home visits may be received by families in different ways. Some families find frequent visits reassuring. Having knowledgeable professionals maintain regular contact reduces the anxiety of sole caregiving responsibility. Other families find frequent visits intrusive and feel that the infant will not truly be "their baby" until they can be autonomous in their caregiving. The family-focused interview, described in Chapter 4: **Maintaining a Family-Centered Approach**, is an excellent opportunity for a family to express their feelings in this regard. The family and the interventionist can work out a visiting plan that is in keeping with the family's goals, with the understanding that this may be later modified.

Coordination With Other Service Providers

Other professionals may also be making home visits to the family. In many communities, a public health nurse or a member of the Visiting Nurse Association may be assigned as part of a high risk infant tracking plan. The team nurse must coordinate with these other professionals so that services are complementary and not redundant. The family's desires about frequency of visits of various professionals should clearly play a role in this coordination.

Further coordination among the various medical specialists following the baby is a role most easily assumed by the team nurse or case manager. In some instances, recommendations by one service provider may conflict with that of another. The family may be confused and frustrated in these situations. A developmental team member may contact the involved specialists, explain the conflict, and get them in touch with each other to work out a solution.

In other instances, one service provider may be unaware of a problem identified by another provider despite the fact that the problem area would usually be seen as an area of responsibility of the former. For example, an infant's poor weight gain may be observed by intervention staff and apnea clinic staff but not by the primary pediatrician. In this case, the family's case manager establishes communication among these service providers to determine who will provide recommendations for and monitor the problem. The ultimate goal is to assist the family in assuming a more active role in resolving these problems. In the period following discharge, however, both the responsibility for caregiving and the medical information are often too new for parents to assume complete autonomy in dealing with discrepancies among recommendations from the various medical specialists. Developmental staff are in a unique position because of their long term relationship with the family to nurture this autonomy.

Another arena for potential conflict revolves around home nursing care. Team members can find themselves in a position to assist families who are receiving home nursing care. Families may experience difficulties in adjusting to nursing care for extended periods in their home. This is not uncommon for families. Home nursing often results in a loss of privacy, and differences in cultural values and practices between the home nurse and the family may arise. Families may need help in identifying and expressing these conflicts. The staff can also help the family in setting reasonable expectations for the nurse's role and in securing agreement from the nursing agency in meeting family expectations. This may be an ongoing process with more than one meeting needed to reach agreement.

Assisting At Risk Families

With the increased incidence of premature delivery among disadvantaged populations, it is common for medically fragile infants to have combined biological and environmental risk status. In some families a variety of factors including teenage motherhood, lack of knowledge, or financial, housing, and transportation problems, may result in poor follow up on needed infant services. When the family has difficulty in keeping medical visit appointments, concern arises as to whether the infant's health status may be jeopardized.

Developmental team members may be in a unique position to play a critical role in these situations in assisting families in keeping appointments and following medical regimens. This may include arranging Medicaid reimbursed taxi service, driving the family directly to the appointment, or agreeing to meet together at the medical visit. In this latter instance, staff may be supportive of the family at a medical visit by helping to communicate and clarify medical information between physician and parent.

Developmental staff can also work to elicit any extended family support that might be available to help the parent follow through on medical needs. Community social service agencies may already be involved with the family, and may also be of assistance in providing the family other support.

In addition, the team's commitment to the family may be demonstrated through bringing formula or toys to the family. Patience and persistence by the team members is also a demonstration of commitment and often will serve in the end to win the family's trust.

DIRECT DEVELOPMENTAL INTERVENTION

The intervention model described in this guide takes into consideration that once discharged from the hospital, some children are unable to access community based intervention programs. Until their medical needs stabilize, this model incorporates the provision of direct physical or occupational therapy and special education services in accordance with the Individual Family Service Plan (IFSP), as described in the previous section. Scheduling of visits within the model is flexible and takes into consideration the family schedule and availability. Initially, the physical or occupational therapist and the special educator may make visits on alternate weeks, or jointly on a weekly basis.

The amount and intensity of intervention typically changes over time. During the early home visits the specialists spend a great deal of time helping the family to make the transition from hospital to home care. The **special educator** helps the family plan a developmentally appropriate environment. This may include suggestions for toys and equipment and for appropriate activities to sustain infant attention and to promote interaction. Direct intervention with the baby is a gradual process and is guided by the baby's signs of readiness. As the infant develops, the educator plans activities to promote attention to objects and social communication.

By the time the infant is discharged, the **physical or occupational therapist** has instituted a program of direct handling to normalize tone and to promote the development of automatic reactions. In the home, the therapist initially recommends therapeutic positions that fit the home environment, and suggests which items of infant equipment are most developmentally appropriate. Caregivers continue to be guided in activities and handling techniques according to the needs of the infant.

The services of the home-based component should be individualized to meet the needs of the family and the infant. Which team member is involved at any specific time should depend upon the family's perceived and stated needs. An analysis of those needs and the services rendered indicated very specific trends of family needs (Long and Baker, 1987). Ten areas of concern and/or need frequently noted by either caregiver or intervention specialist were found in this study. These were grouped into four clusters:

- parent support,
- education,
- motor development, and
- caregiving.

According to the findings, intervention needs change over the infant's first 18 months. *Parent support* and *caregiving information* are most needed by families during the early stages of the infant's life (0-8 months). *Educational development*, especially cognition and language, is of primary concern beginning at about one year of age and continuing through 18 months. Intervention for optimal *motor development* is a consistent need throughout the first 18 months [Table 5].

Table 5

TRENDS IN FAMILY NEEDS
(Long and Baker, 1987)

Age of Infant	Major Developmental Concern
0-8 months	parent support
0-8 months	caregiving information
12-18 months	educational development
0-18 months	motor development

Based on these trends, a family would typically benefit most from intensive support from a **nurse** during the first few weeks at home. Follow up training and support from the nurse eases the transition from the highly supportive NICU environment to home. As the baby's medical condition stabilizes and the family becomes more comfortable with caring for the infant at home, nursing visits can decrease. Most families do not require regular nursing visits after the first four months at home. Though no longer needing to provide technological support and training, the nurse can continue to provide information and assistance regarding feeding, sleeping, and other baby care issues that may be complicated by the medical fragility of the infant.

Developmental intervention may be best delivered by using a holistic approach to the treatment of infants based on a neurodevelopmental philosophy. Because motor needs are a consistent concern, the **physical or occupational therapist** will need to play an ongoing role during the first 18 months. The therapist may need to make continuing weekly visits to provide direct therapy in addition to designing and updating a home program. Additionally, the therapist may need to develop therapeutic strategies that can be integrated with special education goals during the early months.

Parents view **special education** services as increasingly important between 12 and 18 months. By this time, the infant is more medically stable and available for educational interactions. Also, at this time, preterm babies typically begin to show catch-up which helps them assume an active role in the interactions.

Developmental teams committed to the philosophy that parents are the primary caregivers will instruct parents and other caregivers in follow up activities. The primary caregivers are viewed as integral participants during each visit. Explanations of activities and suggestions can be left with the family in a communication book.

During the home based phase, a major thrust is to prepare the infant and family for transition into community based services as soon as possible. Typically this transition occurs between 12 and 24 months. Appropriate community based service models include:

- center based intervention programs,
- home based programs,
- individual therapy, or
- regular day care programs.

Some children who are medically stable, but show indication of a significant handicap, can be assisted in a transition into an intensive daily intervention program prior to 12 months.

Linking the family to community based early intervention programs will allow treatment to be provided in the least restrictive environment, usually within the child's own community. However, in making the decision to assist in the transition to a community based program, family readiness must be taken into consideration. Although the child may show clear signs of readiness for a community based intervention program, the family may be hesitant. Some families find it difficult to give up the support of the hospital team. Others find it difficult to accept their child as handicapped and, thus, in need of a special education program.

Initiating discussion of special education at an early point and continuing to discuss its role can be helpful for the family. Initial resistance to this transition may stem from lack of understanding of the role of special education or individual therapy. In other cases lack of insurance coverage or restrictive health care plans may preclude easy access to individual therapy. It is extremely important, therefore, to explore these issues with the family and to assist them in developing strategies to overcome obstacles.

SUMMARY

In providing services to the families during the home based phase, the ultimate goal of an effective program is to provide appropriate service in the least restrictive environment. Families must be considered integral members of the team in deciding the intensity and the method of the intervention as well as the timing of transitions in intervention programming.

6 INTERVENTION IN THE PICU: MAINTAINING CONTINUITY

In order to provide continuity of developmental services to chronically ill infants, the **PICU** phase is an essential element of the program. In the past, infants and young children who were receiving community-based services often experienced an interruption of services during periods of unstable health and hospitalizations. Developmental teams can now be designed to allow coordinated intervention services to be readily available to these infants while they are hospitalized.

There are usually two groups of chronically ill infants who require services on the PICU during their first two years of life. First, a fairly large number of chronically ill infants require rehospitalization after their initial discharge home. Among the reasons for such rehospitalization are:

- respiratory compromise resulting in poor resistance to upper respiratory infections,
- medical procedures such as tracheostomies or gastrostomies, and
- failure to thrive.

A second smaller group of chronically ill infants require an extremely long initial hospital stay resulting in their transfer directly from the NICU to the PICU when they are four or five months or older. These infants require such long stays because of their extreme prematurity or low birth weight. In a few cases, infants require prolonged hospitalization because of feeding intolerances resulting from short bowel syndrome. Those infants receiving nutrition through a Broviac catheter must often remain in the PICU through most of their first year.

Developmental services should be available to infants who are readmitted to the PICU as well as to those who are transferred directly from the NICU to the PICU. Although both groups of infants and their families need many similar services, there are some specific differences in the intervention provided. These differences will be noted as the PICU services are described in this section.

Prolonged hospitalizations experienced by chronically ill infants can affect the infant's growth and development for a number of reasons. The lack of appropriate stimulation in the hospital, the discomfort of the illness and treatment, the separation from parents, and the interruption of daily routines may pose a threat to the infant's future health and well-being. An infant's illness and hospitalization may also pose problems for parents by interfering with parent-infant attachment and the development of parenting roles (Association for the Care of Children in Hospitals, 1978).

WORKING AS A TEAM

PICU hospitalization requires an interdisciplinary approach with intervention staff working together to provide for both child and family needs. The team nurse can continue in the role of interpreting the infant's medical needs to the parents. Rehospitalizations may necessitate unfamiliar medical treatment resulting in renewed parental anxiety regarding their infant's survival. The developmental team nurse can provide ongoing reassurance and needed explanations regarding conditions that necessitate rehospitalization.

The **special educator** and **physical and occupational therapist** can continue to work together to assure that all of the major developmental needs are promoted to the extent possible during the infant's hospitalization. It is essential that team members integrate their assessment findings and intervention recommendations. The special educator must be aware of positioning and handling techniques that evoke optimal responses from the child. Likewise, the pediatric therapist needs to be aware of the infant's cognitive and psychosocial needs.

Because a hospitalized infant may experience periods of acute distress, interventionists must be sensitive to the infant's capacity for interaction and programming. If weekly staffings are held, the team can discuss the infant's day-to-day tolerance during the acute stage of the illness in order to carefully gradate intervention to the capacity of the infant at any given time. In addition, all interventionists can work together to formulate a developmental plan that schedules intervention sessions at appropriate times. Consideration must be given to the infant's sleep/wake cycle, feeding times, and medical needs.

If hospital-based intervention is to be successful, the nursing staff must be an integral part of the team. The developmental team members must have regular contact with the primary nursing staff to assure that developmental considerations are incorporated into daily caregiving routines. PICU staff can be made aware of developmental needs of the infants using many strategies. For example:

- developmental care plans with positioning diagrams can be displayed at each infant's bedside,
- attendance by developmental staff at patient Rounds facilitates discussion of developmental needs,
- attendance at weekly PICU Child Life Rounds facilitates discussion of family needs, and
- inservice sessions for nurses and residents promotes integration of developmental recommendations into routine caregiving for infants.

FAMILY INVOLVEMENT

An infant's social responsiveness typically provides reinforcement for parents. A hospitalized infant who is socially unresponsive because of medications or illness, provides less social feedback to parents which may diminish their enthusiasm for nurturing the infant. In addition, prolonged or repeated

72

hospitalizations may interrupt the smooth flow of family development and the transition to parenthood. This may, in turn, challenge the parent's sense of competence.

The developmental intervention team will need to be sensitive to family needs arising as a result of the infant's hospitalization. Because feelings of parental competence may diminish during hospitalization, the team members may seek to reassure the family and to promote positive feelings so that infant-parent interactions are not jeopardized. Attendance at Child Life Rounds by developmental staff allows for discussions of family needs with PICU staff. Because of the team's ongoing involvement with the family, they may be able to suggest ways in which the PICU staff may provide support in light of ongoing family issues and concerns.

It is important for a team member to contact the family of a rehospitalized infant as soon as possible after admission to determine the reason for hospitalization and any specific family concerns arising from the hospitalization. This information should be shared with other team members.

Once the infant is settled into the hospital, parents can be encouraged to maintain active involvement with their infant. For example, parents can hold their medically stable infant. Parents sometimes are tentative about holding an infant attached to medical equipment such as IV lines, respirators, and apnea monitors. Team members facilitate parental competence and confidence in handling their hospitalized infant in a variety of ways:

- explaining medical equipment to parents and encouraging them to touch tubes, buttons, etc.,
- showing parents how to manipulate the wires and tubes when holding the infant,
- demonstrating proper handling techniques to calm the infant and to promote the infant's comfort, and
- having the parents hold their infant while the interventionist is present in order to provide them with helpful suggestions and positive reinforcement.

Because families are an important focus of intervention for the team, every effort is made to encourage communication between parents and intervention staff. Since parents often visit their infants at times when developmental staff are not available, the use of a communication book can be instituted. Each parent can receive a *communication book* at the time of their enrollment in the intervention program while their infant is still in the NICU. This book should remain at the baby's bedside.During hospitalization on the PICU, the book can be used for notes between staff and family members to assure ongoing communication. *Phone calls* can also be used to keep parents abreast of their infant's progress, to inquire about how parents are doing, and to respond to family questions. Whenever possible, time should be arranged for the intervention staff to meet the parents during their hospital visits since *face-to-face contact* is always the best method for effective communication.

SPECIAL EDUCATION IN THE PICU

A major goal of the **special educator** is to promote developmentally appropriate activities for the infant during the PICU stay. In order to fulfill that goal, the special educator must function in three roles.

1. *Infant Specialist*--conducting developmental assessments, identifying developmental goals, and providing ongoing intervention in the areas of cognition, self-help, speech, language, and psychosocial development;
2. *Parent Educator*--informing parents of their child's present level of functioning, fostering parental understanding of how hospitalization may affect development, and assisting parents in carrying over developmental activities during hospital visits;
3. *Child Advocate*--actively promoting the incorporation of developmental recommendations into caregiving routines and medical care plans.

The specific steps that the special educator takes in carrying out these roles depend on both the reason for hospitalization and the length of stay.

Short Term Rehospitalization

Before providing special education services to chronically ill infants who are rehospitalized for acute illness or specific surgical procedures, the infant's availability for intervention must be determined. If the infant is found to be medically unstable, the special educator provides nursing staff with background information regarding the infant's typical caregiving routines but does not institute specific developmental activities.

Parents can be encouraged to stay with the infant to provide reassurance and comfort. If the infant tolerates holding, the family can be encouraged to hold the infant whenever appropriate. Because infants are typically accustomed to highly individualized feeding routines, parents should be encouraged to be involved with feeding their infants during their visits. Parents can also be encouraged to bring familiar foods, spoons, pacifiers or bottle nipples to provide their infant with extra comfort and reassurance. Favorite toys from home also provide some familiarity within the environment for the infant. During the short term hospitalization, parents may be able to room in with the infant. The special educator continues in a supportive role to the parents during this particularly anxious time.

Infants experiencing short term hospitalization are often discharged as soon as their health stabilizes. As a result, the special educator's main role consists of providing continuity through the hospital experience and back home again. Once the infant is home, the special educator may determine that the infant has experienced a developmental setback. The original developmental plan may then need to be adjusted appropriately. In addition, home visits by the special educator may need to be increased following discharge from the PICU.

Long Term Hospitalization

Infants who are transferred to the PICU from the NICU and are destined for a prolonged stay on the unit will be in need of ongoing intervention from the special educator. While IFSPs may have been developed during the infant's NICU stay, upon PICU entry a thorough reassessment of the infant developmental functioning will usually be necessary.

Assessment of the infant's functioning in the areas of cognitive, self-help, speech, language, and social-emotional development is completed by the special educator. Because of the special educator's involvement with the infant prior to hospitalization on the PICU, assessment will be enhanced by the familiarity with the individual infant. Assessment is performed during the times when the infant is not in acute distress. The special educator should remain sensitive to the various factors that can impact on the infant's performance. These factors may include the infant's sleep/wake cycle, feeding schedule, and medications.

A variety of assessment instruments can be used by the special educator. The instruments may include the following:

- **Neonatal Behavioral Assessment Scale** (Brazelton, 1984). This scale is a behavioral and psychological exam for the infant between 37 and 44 weeks gestation who is off mechanical support and on room air.
- **Bayley Scales of Infant Development** (Bayley, 1969). This scale provides a measure of the developmental progress of an infant's functioning between two months and two and one half years.
- **Hawaii Early Learning Profile (HELP) Checklist** (Furuno et al., 1984). This developmental checklist facilitates comprehensive individualized assessment, program planning, and recording of child progress in the developmental areas of cognition, language, gross motor, fine motor, social-emotional, and self-help skills. It is used with children from birth to 36 months of age.
- **The Carolina Curriculum for Handicapped Infants and Infants At Risk** (Johnson-Martin et al., 1986). This curriculum provides detailed intervention strategies in the areas of cognition, communication/language, social skills/adaptation, self-help, fine motor, and gross motor functioning. It is appropriate for use with infants with special needs who are functioning in the birth to 24 month developmental age range.

In order to adequately assess the infant, the special educator must be knowledgeable of and comfortable with positioning and handling an infant on medical supports. This may mean working initially with the nursing staff and the physical or occupational therapist to become comfortable handling and positioning the infant before beginning a formal assessment. It may also mean working jointly with nursing staff or therapists during the actual assessment.

The results of the assessment are used to establish developmental goals for the child. Discussion at team staffings can allow the special educator to work with other team members to formulate an overall developmental care plan for the infant. Input from the PICU staff through individual consultation and discussion at weekly Child Life Rounds can also be useful in the development of the plan.

There are two aspects of the *developmental care plan*. First, specific intervention activities generated from the developmental goals should be included in the plan. These activities are carried out by the special educator during sessions with the hospitalized infant. Additionally, strategies intended to be incorporated by the nursing staff and parents during feeding, diapering, bathing and play should also be included in the plan. Discussion with the primary nurse may be needed during the refinement of these strategies.

Communication of the developmental care plan is of utmost importance because the success of the plan depends on its use by many different people. Therefore, a number of strategies for communicating the plan may need to be used. These include:

- activities and positioning suggestions posted at bedside for all caregivers to read,
- a summary of the child's present developmental level and goals noted in the child's medical chart,
- developmental recommendations noted in the parent's communication book, and
- recommendations explained to parents directly whenever possible.

The developmental care plan, therefore, should be directed at nursing and medical staff as well as at the infant's family. Nursing staff can be encouraged to carry out developmental recommendations during their regular caregiving. All efforts should be made to provide recommendations that can be easily incorporated into the infant's routine. A sample plan appears in Figure 13.

Equally important are efforts which are directed at involving the family in developmentally appropriate activities with their infant. Parents should be encouraged to spend as much time with their child as is feasible during a prolonged hospital stay. Participating in feeding, dressing and/or bathing is an excellent way to have parents remain primary caregivers to their infant. Infants typically respond best with their parents and this message is relayed to the parents. By giving parents a positive role in their infant's activities during the hospitalization, parental competence can be fostered. Involvement in routine activities can also help to decrease parental anxieties regarding the infant's medical status by providing parents an active, positive role in meeting their infant's needs.

The hospitalized infant's developmental care plan will usually include intervention activities designed for implementation by the special educator. When the infant is medically stable and tolerates handling by individuals other than primary caregivers, the special educator can institute a regular intervention period. This may occur at least twice a week during which time the special educator implements activities designed to further cognitive, self-help, speech and

Figure 13. Developmental Plan

CHILD DEVELOPMENT CENTER

Developmental Care Plan for: Orlando

Activity

(1) Place musical toys/rattles between Orlando's hands to stimulate gross movement of the arms. Hold the toy slightly off the bed surface so that he will not have to lift it up. Encourage any movement of the arms and hands that is purposeful!

(2) Hold a bright object 10-12" above Orlando's face/chest. Move it <u>slowly</u> back and forth to promote tracking. If he "loses" the object, bring it back for him to find and continue. Start with a horizontal direction and then try vertical!

Position

(1) Place Orlando on his side with a blanket roll along his back to maintain the position. The blanket roll should be between his legs to reduce the stress on the hip joint. His hands should be together toward the midline.

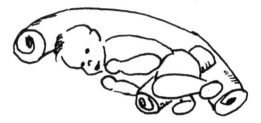

(2) Place Orlando in sitting position. Support a flexed position with blanket rolls. Orlando's head should be in midline with his hands flexed toward his face. Use a towel or blanket roll to prevent his legs from externally rotating and abducting (frog leg position).

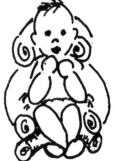

Thanks for helping!

language, and social-emotional goals. The *HELP* and the *Carolina Curriculum* are useful tools to identify appropriate strategies for each identified goal. Initially the infant can be worked with at bedside but may later be transitioned into an infant seat or adaptive equipment, or placed on a floor mat. It is essential for the special educator to work closely with the therapists to assure optimal positioning for the intervention activities.

PHYSICAL/OCCUPATIONAL THERAPY IN THE PICU

The overall goal of therapy in the PICU is to promote optimal *neuromotor development.* In order to accomplish this the therapist must work collaboratively with the medical staff and the special educator to insure that developmental activities are being integrated into the overall care plan of the infant. In addition to directly treating the infant, the therapist must provide input to the nursing staff and parents regarding appropriate motor activities. As with the special educator, the therapist's role with the infant may depend somewhat upon the length of hospital stay and the reason for the hospitalization.

Short Term Rehospitalization

For infants who are rehospitalized for an acute illness or short term medical procedure, the physical/occupational therapist first determines the current neuromotor status of the infant and his/her availability for interaction and handling. The use of a quick neuromotor screening tool such as the *Milani-Comparetti Motor Development Screening Test* (Kliewar, Bruce & Trembath, 1977) provides baseline information on the present status of the infant.

Once the neuromotor status of the infant has been established the therapist can provide the nursing staff with suggestions for positioning and handling the infant. These suggestions may include:

- positions to increase midline orientation, flexion and weight bearing as necessary,
- holding and carrying positions during medical procedures, and
- handling strategies to promote calming or arousal.

Developmental cards can be posted on the crib and notes written in the communication book at each session.

The therapist should encourage the family to continue the program begun at home if it is tolerated by the infant. Maintaining a routine close to that used at home is important for the infant and family. The therapist can work with the special educator and the nurse to encourage this behavior and to support the parents in their attempts.

As the infant becomes more available for interaction, therapeutic intervention can be gradually increased. The therapist can slowly reestablish the degree of handling tolerated by the infant prior to rehospitalization. Alterations in the plan can be made according to the infant's medical status with direct therapy administered only when the infant's medical condition permits.

Long Term Hospitalization

Infants who require long term stays on the PICU can receive direct intervention from the therapist working collaboratively with the special educator and medical staff. Once transferred from the NICU the infant will need an updated assessment to revise the IFSP developed in the nursery.

The physical/occupational therapist will need to reassess the neuromotor status, the developmental skill level, and the oral motor status of the baby. A variety of assessment tools are available to the therapist. In addition to norm-referenced tools, criterion referenced curriculum guides can be utilized in program planning. A sample of instruments that may be used include:

- **The DeGangi-Valvano Test of Motor and Neurological Functions** (TMNF) (DeGangi, Berk, and Valvano, 1983). The TMNF is a neuromotor exam that attempts to quantify the components of the skills usually tested in a traditional neurological exam. Tone is assessed both actively and passively, reflexes are graded according to components rather than simply absence or presence; righting, protective and equilibrium reactions are assessed according to extremity, head and trunk placement.
- **Bayley Scales of Infant Development, Motor Scale** (Bayley, 1969). This scale provides a measure of the developmental progress of infants functioning between two months and 2 1/2 years of age.
- **Subtest of Qualitative Movement Findings** (Valvano and DeGangi, 1986). This structured observation tool used in conjunction with the Bayley Motor Scales allows the therapist to assess the component skills of each developmental task assessed on the Bayley. The tool looks at the posture of the head, trunk, shoulder girdle, pelvis, and extremities during developmental activities. This assists the therapist in program planning and designing treatment strategies.
- **Peabody Developmental Motor Scales** (Folio and Fewell, 1983). This standardized measure of fine and gross motor skills assesses skills from birth to 83 months.

In addition to these specific neuromotor exams, the therapist can also utilize the curriculum guides discussed in the special education section.

Following the reassessment, an updated IFSP can be developed with the family, special educator and the primary medical caregivers. Strategies that are used to reach the goals established in the IFSP include positioning, direct therapeutic handling and the use of adaptive equipment.

Positioning

Proper positioning of the chronically ill infant reinforces the therapist's goals of enhancing flexor patterns, increasing midline orientation and promoting neuromotor organization. Positions discussed under the NICU section remain appropriate for the infant's initial stay in the PICU (Figures 5-8). However, the infant's medical condition dictates readiness for certain positions and tolerance for change. For example, an infant requiring oxygen therapy must not be placed in a position that would compromise respiratory status. Developmental program cards describing the appropriate positions and showing photographs of the infant in these positions are excellent reminders for medical caregivers and family members.

Direct Therapeutic Handling

As the infant's medical condition stabilizes and he or she is able to tolerate direct handling, an ongoing treatment plan can be developed. Using a holistic plan based on neurodevelopmental principles, the therapist can establish a program designed to normalize tone and facilitate developmental skill acquisition and functional skill development. Treatment sessions may be held two to three times per week for 30-60 minutes each. More active participation of the infant during therapy can be facilitated as medical status improves. Games and activities that reinforce treatment objectives can be posted on the crib and in the communication book.

Use of Adaptive Equipment

For the young infant, improved positioning can be achieved simply by the use of blanket rolls. As the infant grows, however, the use of *therapeutic equipment* is sometimes necessary. Providing shoulder support in the infant seat is an initial step in adapting equipment. For the child with lower extremity hypertonicity, additional hip/pelvis stabilization is necessary. The commercially available *Tumble Form Seat* (Preston catalogue) is an excellent seating alternative for the hospitalized infant. To facilitate weight bearing and an upright posture, the use of a *prone stander or supine board* is helpful. A standing schedule is useful in increasing the infant's tolerance for remaining in the apparatus. *Sidelyers, benches, and small tables and chairs* may all prove helpful to carry over treatment goals and objectives. They also provide the infant with alternatives to being in a crib or infant swing. Because of the potential for accidents, the use of baby walkers should be discouraged.

The use and maintenance of adaptive equipment may be an unfamiliar responsibility for most nurses on the PICU. The therapist must work very closely with the nursing staff to encourage consistent use of the equipment and to promote frequent position and equipment changes. Parents can also be helpful in promoting equipment usage. To encourage participation in the long term care plan of the hospitalized infant, it has sometimes been helpful to recruit parents to make or design specific pieces of equipment.

The hospitalized infant's care plan will incorporate a variety of developmental activities. It is important that therapists develop a strong relationship with the medical and nursing staff on the PICU to ensure that the care plan is carried out in a manner that is comfortable for the medical staff and which does not compromise the infant's program or health. Additionally the therapist must collaborate to reinforce the goals and objectives of the IFSP. Parents should be encouraged to participate actively in the care of their infant and be supported in their attempts to do so. Providing an active role for parents is important in fostering competence and decreasing anxiety regarding their ability to care for a chronically ill infant.

DISCHARGE HOME

The ultimate goal of medical and developmental intervention in the hospital is to assure the infant's return home to the family unit. The special educator and therapist work with the developmental team case manager, as discharge nears, to provide a transition to home based programming. The case manager also works with the team nurse regarding provision of medical interventions at home, mobilization of needed home nursing care, and coordination of follow up appointments. The case manager, working with the family, coordinates home visits of the various interventionists following discharge.

7 THE GROUP EXPERIENCE: PROVIDING PARENT-TO-PARENT SUPPORT

While professional support is of undoubted benefit in helping families to cope with the stresses of parenting a medically fragile infant, parents themselves report additional benefits from support from other parents dealing with similar problems (Pizzo, 1983). In the NICU, this support may come from the Parents of Premies organization, Parent-to-Parent organization, or other formal or informal networks developed. Parents' need for support groups vary with the individual needs of the parent and the age of their child. Support groups seem to be especially beneficial when parents are first learning to deal with parenting of a special needs child (Winton and Turnbull, 1981). The parents of an older child may be in a position to provide information and suggestions from the standpoint of "one who has been there" to parents of a medically fragile newborn.

The parent of a medically fragile infant may experience relative social isolation after the infant is at home. This may stem from problems in finding babysitters who can handle the infant's medical needs, not wanting to put the infant in social situations where he or she may be exposed to infections, and just having little time to do things for oneself. These families may benefit from support from peers.

DEVELOPMENT OF THE GROUP FORMAT

Despite the benefits expected from parent-to-parent support groups, designing a format that encourages consistent family participation is often difficult. Meetings held at the hospital, even with provision of babysitters in a room adjacent to the meeting room and reimbursement for transportation costs, may attract only a few families. The authors have found that group meetings that cluster parents in one geographic area are more successful. One parent may be asked to serve as host, with the developmental team making all the arrangements and bringing along all necessary supplies to that parent's home.

Content of the Group

Greater participation may be gained when the sessions are geared as parent-infant activity sessions instead of parent groups. The first 45 minutes can be devoted to group play activities adapted to the level of the participating infants, but which also require participation of the parent. Refreshments can be served after this with the team psychologist providing some open-ended questions related to child management. These may include issues such as development of regular *sleeping patterns*, handling *picky eating behaviors*, and providing appropriate *peer social contact* for the infant. These tend to be issues of shared concern among families so that concerns and possible solutions are readily voiced. These discussions often lead to eliciting broader concerns such as dealing with the uncertainty of the degree of handicap one's child might ultimately have.

Using this format, parents seem more relaxed about sharing concerns than they might in formal hospital-based groups. Friendships of families living relatively near each other are enhanced, prompting some families to get together on their own or to establish phone contact with each other.

Another parent session that has been successful in garnering parent's participation is a *home-made toy workshop* using simple, inexpensive materials. This is especially good in early infancy if mobiles and simple rattles are made. For older infants, some of the techniques used in infant exercise classes employing games with balloons and sheets are fun for parents and infants alike.

Despite the urban location of the chronically ill children served at Georgetown University Hospital, many families described difficulties in finding other nearby children to increase their older infant's social opportunities. Other parents and staff are often able to offer suggestions for finding other families with children. Increasing the community contacts of the family appears to be a widely shared need for parents of medically fragile infants. An additional continuing need is that of respite care and special needs day care, given the large number of working parents.

An attempt was made to examine why a group based at the hospital (a central location to the families) has not always been successful. According to family comments it appears that these families make so many required visits to the hospital that they find it difficult to make a visit that would be more for themselves. Parents seem more willing to participate if they see it as enrichment for the infant. Once in the setting, however, they are quite willing and interested in discussing parenting issues and other sources of concern.

Parent groups serve a useful role in intervention for medically fragile infants. However, to be successful, the group format must be flexible in providing a *time, location and content,* that meets the needs of the families.

CONCLUSION

The complexities of caring for a chronically ill infant require a host of comprehensive services. These infants' overriding medical needs often obscure their need for developmental intervention. Every attempt should be made to maintain continuity in developmental intervention.

With the advent of Public Law 99-457, chronically ill infants will be eligible for developmental intervention from birth. The program described in this guide would appear to be a workable approach to maintaining continuity in intervention on both an inpatient and outpatient basis for infants who remain medically unstable. Intervention programs must be adapted to each hospital setting and staffing pattern. The family-centerd focus in serving chronically ill infants that is described here is timely and in keeping with the mandates of P.L. 99-457. The transactional theory of development would suggest that intervention must be targeted at both the infant and his or her family if we are to see improved outcome for these vulnerable children.

REFERENCES

Als, H. (1984). *Manual for the Naturalistic Observation of Newborn Behavior (Preterm and Full-term Infants.)* Boston: The Children's Hospital.

Als, H. (1986). A synactive model of neonatal behavioral organization: Framework for the assessment of neurobehavioral development in the premature infant and for the support of infants and parents in the neonatal intensive care environment. *Physical and Occupational Therapy in Pediatrics, 6,* 3-53

Als, H., Lawhorn, G., Brown, E., Gibes, R., Duffy, F., McAnulty, G., & Bickman, J. (1986). Individualized behavioral and environmental care for the very low birth weight preterm infant at high risk for bronchopulmonary dysplasia: neonatal intensive care unit and developmental outcome. *Pediatrics, 6,* 1123-1132.

Amiel-Tison, C. (1968). Neurological evaluation of the maturity of newborn infants. *Archives of Diseases of Childhood, 43,* 89-93.

Association for the Care of Children's Health. (1980). *Position statement on critical care for children.* Washington, DC.

Bailey, D. (1987). Collaborative goal-setting with families: Resolving differences in values and priorities for services. *Topics in Early Childhood Special Education, 7,* 59-71.

Bailey, D. & Simeonsson, R. (1984). Critical issues underlying research and intervention with families of young handicapped children. *Journal of the Division of Childhood, 9,* 38-48.

Bailey, D., Simeonsson, R., Winton, P., Huntington, A., Comfort, M., Isbell, P., O'Donnell, K. & Helm, J. (1986). Family-focused intervention: a functional model for planning, implementing, and evaluating individualized family services in early intervention. *Journal of the Division for Early Childhood, 10 (2),* 156-171.

Bennett, F. (1987). The effectiveness of early intervention for infants at increased biological risk. In M. Guralnick and F. Bennett (Eds.), *The Effectiveness of Early Intervention for At-Risk and Handicapped Children* (pp 79-114). Orlando, FL: Academic Press.

Bilotti, G. *Getting children home: Hospital to community.* Washington, D.C.: Georgetown University Child Development Center.

Brazelton, T.B. (1984). *Neonatal Behavioral Assessment Scale,* (2nd ed.). Philadelphia: Lippincott.

Campbell, S. (1983). Effects of developmental intervention in the special care nursery. In M. Wolraich and D. Routh *(Eds.). Advances in developmental and behavioral pediatrics* (Vol. 4, pp. 165-179). Greenwich, CT: JAI Press.

Campbell, S. (1986). Organizational and educational considerations in creating an environment to promote optimal development of high-risk neonates. *Physical and Occupational Therapy in Pediatrics, 6,* 191-204.

Chandler, L., Andrews, M., & Swanson, M. (1980) *Movement assessment of infants: a manual.* Rolling Bay: Washington.

DeGangi, G., Berk, R., & Valvano, J. (1983). Test of motor and neurological functions in high-risk infants: Preliminary findings. *Developmental and Behavioral Pediatrics, 4 (3)*, 182-189.

Dubowitz, L., Dubowitz, V. & Goldberg, C. (1970). Clinical assessment of gestational age in the newborn infant. *Journal of Pediatrics, 77* , 1-10.

Dubowitz, L. & Dubowitz, V. (1981). The Neurological Assessment of the Preterm and Full Term Newborn Infant. *Clinics in Developmental Medicine, No. 79.* Philadelphia: Lippincott.

Ellison, P., Browning, C., & Horn, J. (1983). A large-sample many variable study of motor dysfunction of infancy. *Journal of Pediatric Psychology, 8*, 345-357.

Folio, M. & Fewell, R. (1983). *Peabody Developmental Motor Scales and Activity Cards.* Allen, TX: Teaching Resources.

Furuno, S., Inatsuka, T., O'Reilly, K., Hosaka, C., Zeisloft, B., and Allman, T. (1984). *HELP Checklist (Hawaii Early Learning Profile)* Palo Alto, CA: VORT Corp.

Geik, I., Gilkerson, L., & Sponseller, D. (1982). An early intervention training model. *Journal of the Division for Early Childhood, 5*, 42-52.

Gorski, P., Lewkowicz, D., & Huntington, L. (1987). Advances in neonatal and infant behavioral assessment: Toward a comprehensive evaluation of early patterns of development. *Journal of Developmental and Behavioral Pediatrics, 8*, 39-50.

Hack, M. & Fanaroff, A. (1986). Changes in the delivery room care of the extremely small infant (<750 g.). Effects on morbidity and outcome. *New England Journal of Medicine, 314*, 660-664.

Harris, M. (1986). Oral motor management of the high risk neonate. *Physical and Occupational Therapy in Pediatrics, 6*, 231-253.

Hussey, B. (1988). *Understanding My Signals: Help for Parents of Premature Infants.* Palo Alto, CA: VORT Corp.

Johnson-Martin, N., Jens, K., & Attermeier, S. (1986). *The Carolina Curriculum for Handicapped Infants and Infants at Risk.* Baltimore: Paul H. Brookes Publishing Co.

Kaufman, J. and Lichtenstein, K.A. *The family as care manager: Home care coordination for medically fragile children.* Washington, D.C.: Georgetown University Child Development Center.

Kliewer, D., Bruce, W., & Trembath, J. (1977). *The Milani-Comparetti Motor Development Screening Test.* Omaha, NE: Meyer Children's Rehabilitation Institute, University of Nebraska Medical Center.

Long, T. & Baker, C. (1987, December). *Trends in intervention needs of a group of high risk infants during the first 18 months.* Paper presented at the National Center for Clinical Infant Programs, 5th Biennial National Training Institute, Washington, DC.

Measel, C. & Anderson, G. (1979). Non-nutritive sucking during tube feeding: Effect on clinical course in premature infants. *Journal of Gynecological Nursing, 8*, 265-272.

Morgan, A., Koch, V., Lee, V., & Aldag, J. (1988). Neonatal neurobehavioral examination. A new instrument for quantitative analysis of neonatal neurological status. *Physical Therapy, 68 (69)*, 1352-1358.

Neely, C. (1979). Effects of non-nutritive sucking upon the behavioral arousal of the newborn. *Birth Defects, 15*, 145-171.

Pizzo, P. (1983). *Parent to parent: Working together for ourselves and our children.* Boston: Beacon Press.

Prechtl, H. (1977). Neurological Examination of the Full Term Infant, (2nd ed.) *Clinics in Developmental Medicine, No. 63.* Philadelphia: Lippincott.

Rose, S., Schmidt, K., Riese, M., & Bridger, W. (1980) Effects of prematurity and early intervention on responsivity to tactual stimuli: A comparison of preterm and full-term infants. *Child Development,, 51*, 416-425.

Scull, S. & Dietz, J. (in press). Competencies for the physical therapist in the neonatal intensive care unit. *Pediatric Physical Therapy.*

Shonkoff, J. & Hauser-Cram, P. (1987). Early intervention for disabled infants and their families: A quantitative analysis. *Pediatrics, 80 (5)*, 650-658.

Sweeney, J. (1985). Neonates at developmental risk. In D.A. Umphred (Ed.), *Neurological Rehabilitation*, (pp 137-164). St. Louis: C.V. Mosby.

Valvano, J. & DeGangi, G. (1986). Atypical posture and movement findings in high risk preterm infants. *Physical and Occupational Therapy in Pediatrics, 6 (2)*, 71-85.

Winton, P. & Bailey, D. (1988). The family-focused interview: A collaborative mechanism for family assessment and goal setting. *Journal of the Division of Early Childhood, 12*, 195-207.

Winton, P. & Turnbull, A. (1981). Parent involvement as viewed by parents of preschool handicapped children. *Topics in Early Childhood Special Education, 1*, 11-20.

INDEX